1001 little ways to LOOK YOUNGER

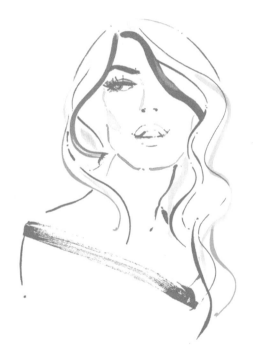

Emma Baxter-Wright

CARLTON BOOKS

THIS IS A CARLTON BOOK

Text copyright © Carlton Books Limited 2007
Design and illustrations copyright © Carlton Books
Limited 2013

This edition published in 2013 by
Carlton Books Limited
20 Mortimer Street
London W1T 3JW

A CIP catalogue record for this book is available
from the British Library.

ISBN: 978-1-78097-254-1

Printed and bound in China

Senior Executive Editor: Lisa Dyer
Designer: Anna Matos Melgaco
Copy Editors: Clare Hubbard and Diana Craig
Illustrator: Kerrie Hess
Production: Maria Petalidou

This book reports information and opinions
which may be of general interest to the reader.
Neither the author nor the publisher can accept
responsibility for any accident, injury or damage
that results from using the ideas, information or
advice offered in this book.

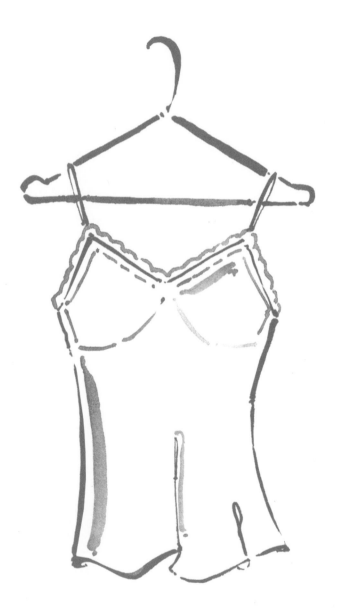

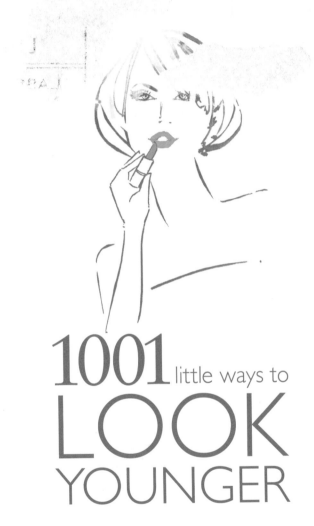

1001 little ways to
LOOK
YOUNGER

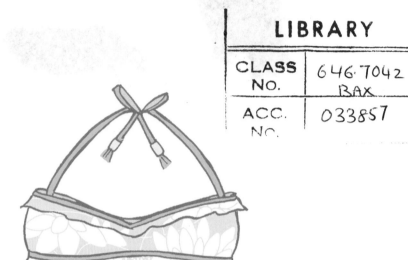

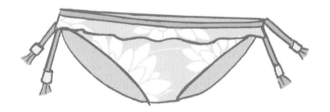

CONTENTS

INTRODUCTION

Did you know it's possible to reduce a saggy jawline simply by exercising your facial muscles, that eating a diet rich in EFAs will make your skin glow, and that getting a good night's sleep is vital for physical regeneration?

Although it's not possible to stop the clock from ticking and halt the ageing process, there are hundreds of little things you can do to slow it down. From cosmetic surgery to simply making daily life changes, it is possible to prevent damage and reverse the external signs of ageing. Here we've gathered together 1001 tips to help you make the most of what you've got and help you look and feel years younger.

Top ten ways to look younger

15
KEEP ON DRINKING
(see Skincare, page 11)

180
USE SPF 30 EVERY DAY
(see Skincare, page 48)

273
WHEN TO COVER THE GREY
(see Hair Care & Styling, page 68)

SKINCARE

understanding your skin

1 FIGHT FREE RADICALS

Free radicals, small unstable oxygen molecules, attach to other cells of the body and break them down. The skin protein collagen is particularly susceptible to free radicals, which cause the collagen molecules to break down and re-link up a different way, which in turn makes them become stiff and less mobile. Eating foods rich in antioxidants and using skin products that contain antioxidants can help reduce free radicals.

2 KEEP HYDRATED

With age, cells stop regenerating at the rate they once did and in the same efficient way. Cells become more abnormally shaped, which makes the texture of the skin appear different and prevents the skin from retaining water. As a result, the skin's texture and water-retaining ability is diminished. The recommended daily intake of water is 2.2 litres (75 fl oz) a day for women and 3 litres (100 fl oz) for men.

3 FAT LOSS MAKES YOU LOOK OLDER

As you age the underlying supportive fat tissues decrease, facial muscles become more slack and bone deteriorates, so the structure on which the skin sits becomes weaker. Younger people have more fat cells, as do those carrying more weight, which is why many larger, older people have fewer wrinkles.

4 STOP THE CAUSES OF SKIN AGEING

Knowing all the possible causes of premature skin ageing can help you take preventative action. The main culprits are free-radical damage to our cells from exposure to the sun, cigarette smoke, toxins and pollution, but poor diet, excessive alcohol consumption, stress, sleep deprivation and the use of harsh skin products can all accelerate the process.

5 SPOT YOUR TYPE OF SKIN AGEING

Chronologically aged skin is a result of natural internal factors and manifests as thinner and less elastic skin that is otherwise smooth and unblemished. Photo-aged skin, however, is marked by wrinkles, age spots, uneven pigmentation and a more leathery appearance.

6 IDENTIFY YOUR SKIN TYPE

In order to choose the right skincare products, you need to know your skin type. Dry skin usually has an uneven skin tone, visible capillaries and flakiness, while oily skin is more prone to visible pores, breakouts and areas of pigmentation.

7 SKIN CHANGES

The texture of skin alters frequently depending on environmental factors like pollution and weather so you should change your skin products accordingly. To check up on the current state of your skin, hold a magnifying mirror up close to your cleansed face in bright daylight and look for identifying clues.

improving your habits

8 SPOIL YOURSELF

As you get older it's important to indulge yourself with regular facials. Women who work hard at being beautiful believe there are no ugly women in the world, just ones that get neglected. If your skin feels great, you feel beautiful all over.

9 PILLOW PRESSURE

Burying your face in a pillow puts pressure on your skin, which reduces circulation. Over time, the wear and tear this causes will break down collagen and cause lines and wrinkles. Switch to silk, satin or a high thread count cotton to minimize the friction on facial skin.

10 SLEEP AWAY WRINKLES

Keep your neck stretched upwards by sleeping on a high-density contour foam pillow that conforms to your shape and provides maximum support. It will help prevent sleep wrinkles from forming on your face and neck.

11 STOP SMOKING

Smoking tobacco changes the skin's DNA repair process, leading to the breakdown of collagen and elastin fibres and resulting in premature lines and wrinkles. It also starves the skin of oxygen and essential nutrients and severely dehydrates it, all of which causes premature ageing.

12 AVOID SMOKY AREAS

Stay out of places where you will be exposed to other people's smoke. Some researchers believe that exposure to cigarette smoke in a confined area is as bad for your skin as the sun's ultraviolet rays. The smoke has a drying effect on the skin's surface plus it restricts blood vessels, so reducing blood flow and depleting oxygen. Even passive smoking will deplete vitamin C, a key ingredient for keeping skin plump and moist.

13 BREAK BAD HABITS

Any repetitive movement such as chewing gum, frowning or sucking on a cigarette will lead to the development of fine lines. Over time micro-tears will appear in the skin resulting in collagen-damaging inflammation. The physical act of smoking causes you to squint, and exaggerates wrinkles around the eyes. It also relies on the repetitive action of pursing your lips: every time you suck in, the small wrinkles around your mouth become bigger.

14 PERFECT SLEEPING POSTURE

Sleeping curled up on your side in the foetus position will create wrinkles and creases on the side of your face where the skin is at its thinnest. Try to sleep on your back at night (and avoid rolling over to dribble into the pillow), if you want to wake up with a smooth and crease-free face.

15 KEEP ON DRINKING

Drinking at least 6 glasses of water a day will to help suppress the appetite, metabolize fat and keep your body and skin fully hydrated and younger-looking. Diet Coke, herbal teas and fruit juice will not provide the same benefits to your body as plain water.

cleansing

16 CLEANSE ACCORDING TO SKIN TYPE

One thing all dermatologists agree on is that you should use the right products for different skin types. Dry skin should be cleansed without removing the skin's protective film so you need a thick, milky cleanser. Oily skin needs oil-based products as they dissolve sebum effectively. For normal skin, try anything gentle and water-based.

17 FRESH-FACED GLOW

If you mix a tiny blob of exfoliating cream with your nightly cleanser, you will have a fabulous fresh face that looks smooth and glowing the following morning, with the impurities drawn out.

18 SHORT SHOWERS

A combination of water that is too hot, and washing your face and body with soap will dissolve the skin's natural moisture balance, so keep your daily shower short and water temperature moderate if you want to avoid dry skin.

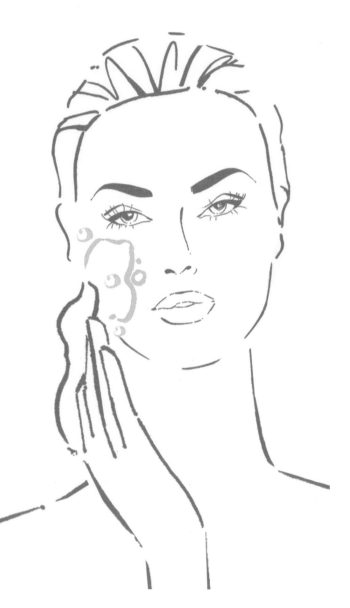

19 QUICK AND EASY CLEANSING

There are many facial wipes on the market to help speed up the cleansing process, but make sure you choose the correct one for your skin. Many are formulated for teenagers and are too harsh for older skin. Even the antiageing varieties can be quite harsh, so go for wipes for sensitive skin.

20 HANDS OFF

Always resist the urge to poke and prod blackheads and pimples. Even the smallest spot can flare up, and what started as a minor blip on the landscape can turn into a pea-sized crater. Use a small blob of calendula cream for babies overnight to dry it up.

21 CLEAN UP BEFORE BEDTIME

Older skin needs more TLC than a teenager's, so never ever go to bed without removing your make-up, which will clog up the pores and stop your skin from breathing, promoting the growth of blemishes and blackheads in the morning. You also have more time in the evening than the morning to devote to skincare – so make it a habit.

creams, serums & moisturizers

22 WATER WORKS WONDERS

Kickstart the active ingredients in all skincare products by applying them to skin that is a little damp. Run wet hands over your face or body before putting on wrinkle creams or cellulite serums, and not only will they start working immediately but they will also penetrate the outer layer of skin more easily.

23 IS IT WORKING?

If you are unsure about the effectiveness of your antiageing products, cut right back on the number of products you are using. Most people use far too many different ones, which makes it difficult to assess their efficiency. In addition to your usual day and night moisturizers, try just one other wrinkle cream for a week to see if there are any beneficial results.

24 REPLACE OLD PRODUCTS

Skin creams with active ingredients have a shelf life so don't expect them to last forever. Once a month sweep all free samples and airport purchases off your shelves, and decide to invest only in products that are targeted at your age and skin stage.

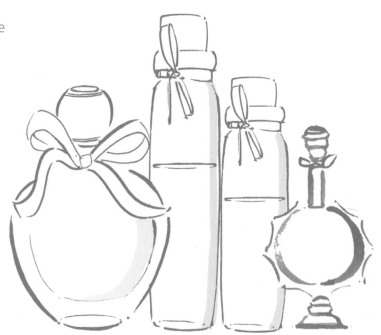

25 BUMPY SKIN

Overloading products can lead to congested pores and tiny rough bumps all over your skin. To keep skin hydrated and smooth, reduce the number of lotions and creams you are using, and instead use a resurfacing treatment once a week, along with a good-quality SPF daily moisturizer.

26 PRODUCT PLACEMENT

Be careful about laying one product on top of another and overloading your skin. Too many different ingredients and too much actual 'lotion' can result in irritation and over-sensitized skin.

27 NIGHT REPAIR WORK

The skin repairs itself most effectively between the hours of 1 am and 3 am, so products aimed at addressing blemishes and eruptions will be more effective overnight. Use an acid-based night-time skincare product after cleansing to exfoliate the outer layers of skin and hydrate the deeper layers.

28 BREATHE DEEP

Make your replenishing night cream more effective by taking five deep breaths to boost levels of oxygen to the skin before smoothing on your cream.

29 SERUM COMES FIRST

A serum that contains 'active' ingredients for a specific purpose is usually applied to the skin before a moisturizer. As these products are very intensive, only a few tiny drops are needed, so it is worth investing in the best you can afford. As skin ages and produces less sebum it needs daily moisturizing, so you can use both products for a combined result.

30 FIGHT CITY POLLUTION

Urban pollution plays havoc with your skin. Windborne dust, particles of dirt and smog can all clog up your pores and make your skin choke. Use a daily moisturizer that is specially formulated for city skin to act as a barrier against pollution. Don't forget to cleanse thoroughly at the end of the day.

31 LOOKING FOR RADIANT SKIN

Facial brighteners are a new antiageing product. They target cells in the epidermis that have become hardened and lost their ability to reflect pink tones of light. Brighteners amplify full-scale reflectivity and bring a fresh luminescence to the skin.

32 SERIOUS ABOUT SERUMS

Older skin benefits from the use of serums, which contain targeted ingredients to help tone and lift the skin. These products can penetrate the epidermis in a deeper way than moisturizers because they have a smaller molecular structure.

33 FIRM UP WISELY

Firming face creams are ideal for skin that has become saggy and lost its natural elasticity because the cream temporarily tightens as well as moisturizes. They usually contain hyaluronic acid to help rebuild collagen and create a firmer foundation.

34 SOFTEN STRETCHMARKS AND WRINKLES

Marketed as a miracle cream version of Botox that relies on peptid technology (which helps photo-aged skin and is claimed to perform better than vitamin C or retinol), Strivectin was originally used to improve the appearance of stretchmarks. Although no cream can relax wrinkles away, there is some evidence that Strivectin may help prevent new lines forming and reduce the deepness of existing wrinkles.

35 MOISTURIZE BEFORE MAKE-UP

Apply moisturizer before you put on your make-up because it will give the skin a healthy, plumped-up look. Wait 5–10 minutes and then apply your make-up over the moisturizer.

36 SAFEGUARD SENIOR SKIN

As we get older, the skin on our face starts to get thinner and drier. It needs extra protection and lots of moisturizing cream, especially in the cold winter months. Avoid harsh toners, and replenish lost hydration with a firming face cream.

skincare ingredients

37 ANTI-INFLAMMATORY AID

New antiageing products are packed full of ingredients that are used as anti-inflammatories. Deep-set lines and wrinkles are being treated like wounds with new 'healing' creams.

38 PREVENTATIVE SKINCARE

To counteract potential future damage, top dermatologists recommend you look for the following antioxidants in your daily moisturizer: idebenone, ferulic acid, vitamins C and E, coenzyme Q10 and lycopene.

39 SEARCH OUT 'ACTIVE' INGREDIENTS

By law, the first ingredient listed on a label should have the highest concentration in the formula. The term 'active' means an ingredient that works beneath the skin's surface to produce visible changes. For it to work, however, it has to be protected from air and light, and used regularly.

40 C IS FOR COLLAGEN

Vitamin C is essential in both face creams and diet because it is necessary for the formation of collagen, the protein that gives skin its elasticity and strength. As an antioxidant it destroys harmful free radicals in the body, caused by pollution, stress and a poor diet. If unchecked, these attack the skin and lead to premature ageing.

41 CHOOSE KIWI FOR THE SKIN

As well as vitamins C and E, potassium and magnesium, kiwi fruit contains high concentrations of alpha-linolenic acid which helps retain moisture in the skin and hair. Kiwi seed oil contains more than 60% of ALAs, making it ideal for skin products.

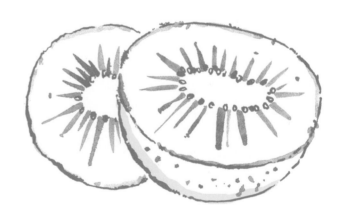

42 MAGIC MUSHROOMS

Fermented extract of the Kombucha mushroom is a new treatment for the face, promising to multiply the production of collagen in skin cells, which in turn will plump up the skin and generally improve its appearance.

43 LOOK FOR PRO-PEPTIDES

Long known for their effectiveness in treating damaged skin, peptides are now thought to help reduce fine lines and wrinkles. They can help stimulate the production of collagen and hyaluronic acid in the skin's upper layers, which is vital in the support structure of the skin which breaks down as we age.

44 FRANKINCENSE IS A WISE CHOICE

Look for this ingredient in organic skincare products; the sweet light oil has long been famous for its purifying properties, and in cream forms it is used for soothing and toning and as a skin repairer in antiageing products.

45 WONDER VITAMIN

When skin begins to look dull and lifeless vitamin A can provide assistance. Found in retinol, tretinoin, tazarotene and palimate (new developments are on the way) it increases skin elasticity and dermal thickening and reverses photo-ageing.

46 MIRACLE IN A JAR

Alpha-lipoic acid is a potent antioxidant that can help repair existing skin damage and fight future damage, because it is soluble in both oil and water, which permits its entrance to all parts of the cell. It diminishes fine lines and gives skin a healthy glow.

47 THE A LIST

Retinoids are the synthetic version of vitamin A, the first generation of which are called Retin-A, and retinol. They have been shown to have fantastic results in treating wrinkles and spotty skin, as they increase the turnover of cell growth and regenerate new skin.

48 TRY TAZAROTINE

Although only available on prescription at the moment, British scientists think tazarotine and tretinoin (whose active ingredient is related to vitamin A) can effectively reduce visible wrinkles, especially those caused by sun damage.

49 SKIN-SAVING ANTIOXIDANT E

Vitamin E is known to be one of the most powerful antioxidants, which can help prevent free radical damage caused by environmental factors like the sun. It is found in more and more skin creams to help ward off this damage, but you can source it nutritionally from leafy green vegetables and olive oil.

50 CREAMY COPPER PEPTIDE

When added to skin creams, copper peptides combine with other enzymes in the body, and have been shown to promote collagen and elastin production. They can help to reverse the ageing process by thickening the skin and reducing fine wrinkles.

51 SOOTHE IT WITH OILS

Lavender is the most versatile essential oil, good for helping general fatigue and tension as well as easing skin irritations. Neroli oil, distilled from the leaves of the bitter orange tree, can help balance both oily and dry skin, while sandalwood is a wonderfully balancing oil that can also help soothe skin irritations.

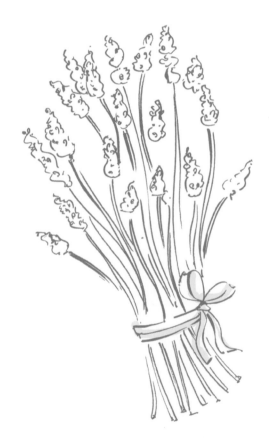

52 WRINKLE FIGHT WITH MALACHITE

The exquisite green mineral is thought to be a powerful tool in the antiageing battle. The mineral increases cellular water retention, giving the complexion a temporary tighter, firmer appearance.

53 KINETIN SKINCARE

Keep an eye out for skincare products that contain the plant growth hormone kinetin (N6-furfuryladenine), which has been shown to have dramatic effects on ageing skin, helping to improve the appearance of fine lines and wrinkles, and reduce blotchiness.

54 A NATURAL ANTIDOTE TO MATURING

The production of hormones in the body declines with age, which results in everything starting to dry out, especially the skin. Look for wrinkle creams with phyto-oestrogens called isoflavones, which mimic the effect of the female hormone oestrogen and will help to keep skin hydrated and toned.

55 SOMETHING FISHY

Skincare products containing DMAE (dimethylaminoethanol) show good results in the reduction of fine lines and wrinkles. Source it naturally by eating more fish, such as anchovies and sardines which contain high concentrations.

56 PAPAYA PICK-ME-UP

Look out for papaya enzyme peel, which uses the natural fruit enzyme papain to give your skin the same smooth fresh feel as an AHA (alphahydroxy acid) treatment but without the harsh chemicals.

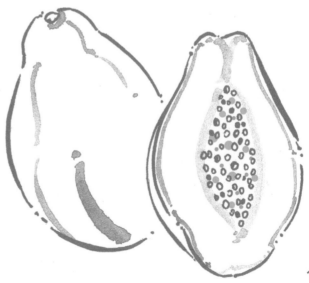

exfoliators & polishers

57 BE A GENTLE SCRUBBER

Older skin needs careful treatment. Keep your exfoliation routine gentle and look for a product that has spherical grains that won't scratch your skin. Always exfoliate on damp skin. Gentle rubbing in a circular movement for a maximum of two minutes will remove dead skin and encourage fresh new cells to flourish.

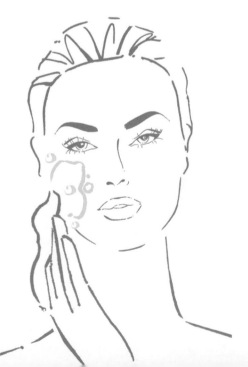

58 NEW CELLS, NEW SKIN

Young skin renews itself every month. As we get older, the process slows down, so gentle exfoliation will help to maintain the cycle of renewal, scrubbing away dead cells and leaving you with smooth skin – but keep the treatment to once a week.

59 NON-ABRASIVE RETEXTURIZING

Don't be tempted to use a body scrub on the delicate skin of your face. Good-quality face exfoliators use calibrated diamond-shaped crystals for precision removal of dead skin cells from the epidermal layer. Body scrubs contain larger, rougher granules that will irritate and inflame sensitive faces.

60 NATURAL VERSUS SYNTHETIC

Natural abrasive scrubs like walnut kernels work best on younger skins. Synthetic options commonly found in microdermabrasion creams contain particles that are smooth and spherical. Especially designed for older skin, they will not cut or scratch it.

61 LOOK OUT FOR AHAS

Traditionally based on natural acids derived from fruit and plants, alphahydroxy acids (AHAs) are now manufactured synthetically. They act as a mild exfoliant by dissolving the 'glue' that binds skin cells together, thus allowing old cells to be shed in favour of new young ones. Non-abrasive, they are available in exfoliating creams or masks.

62 SEARCH OUT SALICYLIC ACID

This is the only betahydroxy acid that works mainly as an exfoliant to improve the skin's colour and texture. It is an oil-soluble acid that can penetrate into the pores that contain sebum, and exfoliate the dead skin cells that build up inside.

63 ABRASIVE OVERDOSE

Don't overdo the exfoliating treatments. Dermatologists have seen a rise in the number of patients coming in for help after too-harsh therapies. After the age of 35, you need to focus on the protection and maintenance of your skin rather than correcting it.

64 REFINE WITH A PORE MINIMIZER

Specially formulated cleansers to reduce the appearance of large pores usually do so via a thermal warming agent, which opens the pores. The cream has inbuilt cleansers and exfoliators that clean and slough away the debris and tighten the skin, for a more refined appearance.

65 BRIGHT AND BEAUTIFUL

Over-the-counter purifying peels can have excellent results. A two-step kit will start with an exfoliating antibacterial wash that contains tiny particles of pumice stone to slough up the skin. The peel solution is then left on overnight and washed off in the morning for visibly brighter skin.

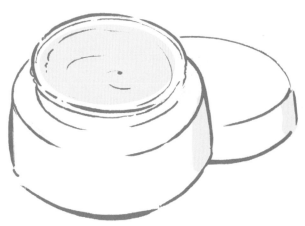

66 DIY DAMAGE

Treat your skin gently, as the older you are, the thinner it gets. Vigorous rubbing during exfoliation or microdermabrasion treatments will increase its sensitivity and lead to a loss of pigmentation.

67 POLISH YOUR OWN SKIN

Exfoliants and microdermabrasion treatments will slough away layers of dead skin cells to leave fresh unblemished skin that glows with vitality. Gentle exfoliation will help to erase fine lines and wrinkles, as well as stimulating oil production and circulation, which in turn encourages new skin cells to grow.

68 SKINCARE THAT'S SCIENTIFIC

Many products contain alphahydroxy acids (AHAs), which are derived naturally from sugars in plants. They work because they have molecules small enough to penetrate the outer layer of the skin, and reach the lower layer. They also dissolve the cement that holds dead skin cells together, increasing cell turnover, and sloughing off dull, rough skin on the surface.

face treatments

69 ZAP NEW FREE RADICALS

New studies show that mobile phones and computers emit electromagnetic waves that can penetrate the skin. Protect your skin with Expertise 3P, a skin-fortifying mist with plant extracts that helps the cell walls stay intact.

70 COLD SPOON COMPRESS

For a quick fix for puffy eyes, keep two metal teaspoons in the fridge. Place the metal on the swollen area and gently press for at least 60 seconds to reduce any puffiness.

71 MAGNETIC FACELIFT

Promising to smooth out wrinkles and deliver a boost to ageing skin, a magnetic face mask consists of 19 magnets, which are strategically placed on the face. For any improvement to be noticed, the magnets need to be used for between 30 and 60 minutes a day for at least a couple of weeks.

72 STIMULATE COLLAGEN PRODUCTION

Facial acupuncture is thought to give you clearer, brighter skin. It is also believed to stimulate collagen fibres, resulting in increased elasticity of skin, as well as plumping out wrinkles.

73 NEVER EXPERIMENT ON THE DAY

Face masks, skin bleaching, soothing eye pads or any other beauty procedure that will affect the way your skin looks should not be carried out for the first time immediately prior to a special occasion. Even 'normal' skin can turn red and lumpy, so only experiment on quiet nights when your social calendar is free.

74 THE DO-NOTHING FACELIFT

Retrain your face muscles to assume their correct, relaxed and natural appearance with stick-on 'Frownies'. Designed to be worn overnight on the forehead and between the brows, they work to smooth underlying facial muscles and so reduce expression lines, leaving younger-looking skin.

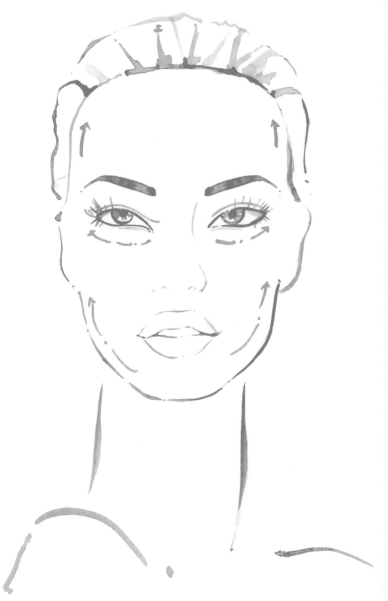

23

75 TROPICAL FACE MASK

The common coconut has fantastic benefits for more mature skin. Cut up the flesh in a blender, then add boiling water and process for 10 minutes. Finally, squeeze the resulting mixture through cheesecloth. Coconut helps to prevent free radical formation, and penetrates the connective tissues to keep them strong and supple.

76 PRE-PARTY PREP

Prior to a big event, choose a 'lifting' and lymphatic drainage-based treatment, which will improve the appearance of skin tone and reduce puffiness, rather than one that deals with extractions, which is more likely to bring impurities to the surface and may cause your skin to break out.

77 30-SECOND SKIN REVIVER

Place a fresh hand towel into steaming hot water (not boiling) and then cover your entire face with it for 30 seconds. Use the flannel to buff the T zone area, chin, nose and forehead, and then splash freezing cold water all over your face to leave pores tight and tingling.

78 SWEET AS HONEY

Once a week, apply a honey face mask for 30 minutes. It is nourishing for the skin, and will leave your skin soft and supple. Simply apply honey straight from the jar onto skin that has been moistened with warm water. Rinse off with warm water, then splash with cold water to close the pores.

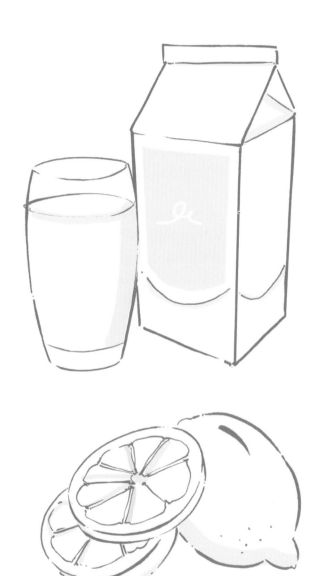

78 FACIAL ACUPUNCTURE

In facial acupunture, tiny needles are inserted all over the face to clear blocked energy in your body and alleviate stress, which causes wrinkles. The treatment aims to clear blockages and restore balance so that the body functions efficiently and skin looks healthy and radiant.

80 SPA TREATMENT AT HOME

This light therapy system stimulates collagen and elastin production and helps to diminish fine lines. The machine has two panels of visible red and infrared light, which penetrate the skin with pulses of non-thermal light energy, triggering a response from the skin. The treatment takes 10 minutes a day.

81 KITCHEN SKIN BRIGHTENER

Dull and sallow skin will benefit from equal measurements of lemon juice and milk mixed together and worked gently into a clean face with a soft bristled cosmetic brush. Leave for 5 minutes before rinsing off for brighter, tingly skin.

82 PLUG IN FOR A FACIAL

Using a micro-current machine, the CACI facial treatment carefully massages the muscles in the face using tiny electric impulses that gently exercise the delicate muscles, leaving skin lifted and tighter.

83 FRESHEN UP

If your skin looks dull and stressed, spritz on chilled rose water to instantly revitalize and freshen up. Follow this with a moisturizing rose facial oil massaged into the skin with small circular movements. This will boost circulation and promote a healthy glow.

84 A FRESH AIR FACIAL

An oxygen facial targets the face to improve the appearance of the skin using the latest biotechnology. Pure oxygen mist is blasted into the basal layer of the skin to deliver antioxidants, boost circulation and revive a tired and sallow complexion.

85 THREAD VEINS ON CHEEKS

Horse chestnut cream is said to strengthen the tiny red veins that appear on the cheeks and nose when skin becomes thinner and loses some of its collagen. It's also available in tablet form to help boost general blood circulation in the skin.

86 HYDROQUINONE ON PRESCRIPTION

Often called lightening creams, products containing hydroquinone are used to treat age spots and hyperpigmentation. Hydroquinone works by blocking the production of the pigment melanin during the skin's natural exfoliation process. It is available in over-the-counter products, but a stronger formula can be prescribed by your doctor or dermatologist.

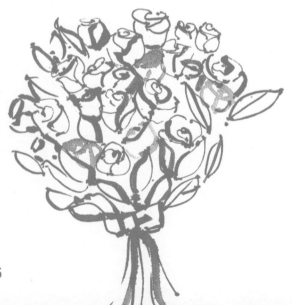

87 FADE AWAY

To treat small areas of uneven pigmentation and age spots, look for products containing both kojic acid and hydroquinone. Used as a night-time treatment and massaged gently into the skin, these natural lighteners reduce discoloration.

88 WAKE UP WITH WATER

To revive tired skin each morning, splash cold water all over your face. It will cause your skin to contract, leaving it fresh and tingly, as well as boosting circulation and making you feeling energized.

89 TWO MINUTE FACE-LIFT

A simple egg white and lemon juice face mask that you whip up in the kitchen has a tightening effect on the skin, and will leave it feeling fresh and glowing.

90 AVOCADO PICK-ME-UP

Take a ripe avocado and simply place slices of it onto your skin, particularly on the very dry parts. Older skin becomes drier and more translucent, and the oil within the fruit will activate increased oil production within your skin, giving you a softer and younger look.

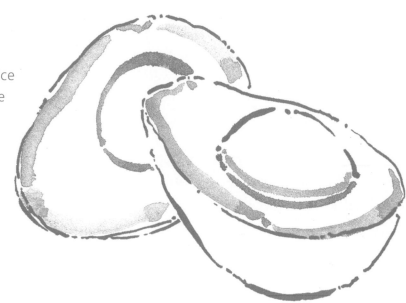

facial exercise & massage

91 WOBBLY CHIN BE GONE

A quick-fix facial toner that can be repeated 20 times a day wherever you are is to push your lips tightly together and make a wide grimace. Hold for 3 seconds and repeat, to contract lower facial muscles and tighten a wobbly chin.

92 TIGHTEN UP FACIAL MUSCLES

Like a wobbly tummy, facial muscles need to be exercised on a regular basis to stop them becoming loose and flabby. A routine that takes just 10 minutes a day, and which can be done anywhere – on the bus, in the car or watching TV – will tighten up lazy skin.

93 PLUMP YOUR MOUTH WITH A BAND

Try a facial flex fitness device specifically for facial muscles. Just two minutes a day with a resistance band should improve circulation and skin firmness, and help to reduce double chins and a wrinkly jaw.

94 GET YOUR FINGERS WORKING

Just a few minutes a day of fingertip massage can increase circulation in the face, leaving your complexion revitalized and rigid frown lines less set. Age causes the connective tissue to become less supple, so massage must be delicate and fingers not probe too deeply. Try simply tapping two fingers from beside the mouth to along the jawline to stimulate circulation and promote glow.

95 PINCH TO RELIEVE STRESS

Many people hold stress in the area between the brows and, in time, vertical stress lines will develop. When you feel your brow knit together with concentration or stress, take a moment to pinch the muscle here, working from the centre of the brow along the browline in each direction with a thumb and bent forefinger.

96 MASSAGE WITH A FRIEND

Regular facial massages don't have to mean an expensive trip to the salon – it is the action of gentle massage on the face that relaxes the muscles, stimulates the blood vessels under the skin and helps keep fine lines at bay.

97 WAKE UP YOUR FACE

In the morning, the face can look pale and puffy because of the natural nocturnal slow-down in the body. When putting on your moisturizer, take the opportunity to gently massage all the muscles in the face to waken up the lymphatic system and jumpstart the circulation.

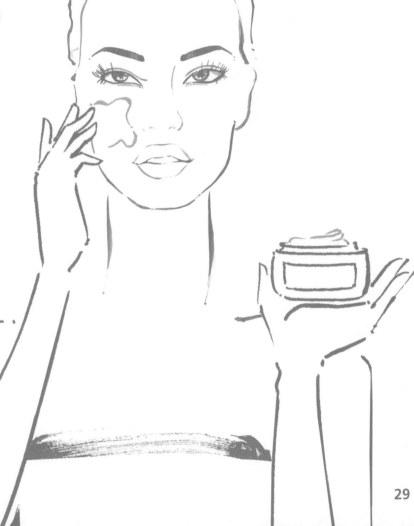

eye care

98 ESSENTIAL EYE CARE

The skin around our eyes has a tendency to get fine lines and wrinkles because there are no oil glands in the skin directly beneath and above the eyes. You should always use a cream designed just for that area, to keep skin moisturized. Put four drops of cream under each eye from below the pupil to the outer corner at the crow's-feet and pat into place.

99 ONE-SHOT WONDER

An innovative new gel called Laresse is available for small eyebrow creases, and wrinkly crow's-feet. Made in the lab rather than from human or animal sources, it has been praised for its super-smooth results.

100 HERBAL TREATMENT

Reduce puffy or swollen eyes with a green tea compress. Dip cotton wool into the green tea, drain off excess moisture, then dab gently around the eye area. This will help to tighten the skin around the eyes.

101 SMOOTH FINE EYE LINES

After a night out in a smoky atmosphere, eyes can become tired and red. Soothe them by grating cucumber onto a muslin cloth. Wrap it up like a tortilla wrap and hold it gently against your eyes. The enzymes in the cucumber will help to reduce swelling and smooth out fine lines.

102 WAKE UP WITH REFRESHED EYES

Keep a bottle of toning eye make-up remover in the fridge, and use the solution to gently clean your eyes in the morning. The chilled remover will help de-puff the eyes as well as clean.

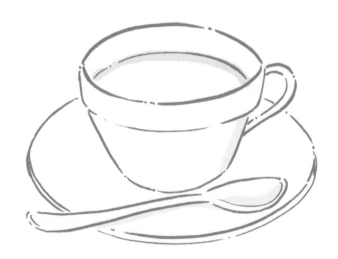

103 STRENGTHEN UNDER-EYE CAPILLARIES

Some under-eye creams, such as Hylexin, contain ingredients that are meant to help strengthen the capillaries that leak blood under the eyes and cause the dark black and blue tints. Make sure the formulas include ingredients that support elastin and collagen too, as these will help firm the skin and improve its ability to 'spring back'.

104 GENTLY DOES IT

Removing make-up before bedtime should be done with an oil-based make-up remover using a small cotton wool pad and cotton buds (Q-tips) Clean the delicate area around the eye and up to the brows by dabbing gently without rubbing.

105 PAD YOUR EYES

There are several under-eye beauty pads on the market that contain powerful botanicals, such as soybean extracts, to temporarily reduce puffiness and dark circles after a week. They are contoured to the under-eye area. You will need to wear them for 30 minutes a day to see results.

106 DRINK TO BANISH DARK CIRCLES

Improving your circulation and keeping your body hydrated by drinking water throughout the day will help reduce the appearance of dark circles under your eyes. Solving the problem this way, through a healthy practice, will produce longer-lasting results than trying to disguise it with cosmetics, which gives only a short-term fix.

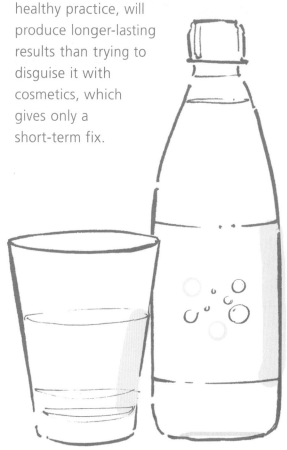

107 DE-PUFF EYES WITH MASSAGE

Using small circular motions of fingers on the face, you can help clear the lymphatic drainage system and de-puff tired eyes and skin. Massage away from the centre of your face in a symmetrical way – from forehead to temples, nose to ears and chin to jawbone – using facial oil.

108 EXTRA PILLOWS

If you have time in the morning, slip an extra pillow under your head for 15 minutes before you get up. Lie quite still and let gravity drain the fluid from your eye bags, for a fresh-faced way to start the day.

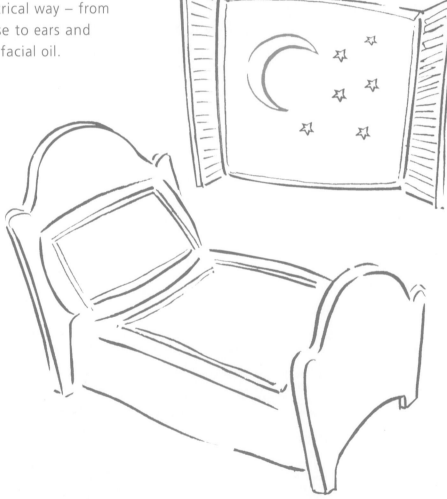

neck & bust

108 BRISK STROKES UPWARDS

Use a pro-collagen lifting product to prevent premature ageing of the neck. Apply using alternate hands in a brisk upwards action, starting below the collarbone, to help improve skin tone.

110 BUST-FIRMING CURRENTS

The Ionithermie bust-firming treatment uses a combination of thermal clay and algae, which is spread over the chest. Two types of electric current are then alternated through this layer, to tone and support the muscles around the breast area, visibly lifting the bust.

111 FERULIC ACID FOR PHOTODAMAGE

The décolletage is very prone to photo-ageing, so protect it with a serum that contains ferulic acid (a natural antioxidant that most plants produce). This is particularly beneficial for skin suffering from redness (erythema) or which is photodamaged or hyperpigmented.

112 LOVE BEHIND YOUR EARS

Always remember to use antiageing serums and moisturizer behind your ears and the back of your neck, to keep your hidden areas well hydrated and help prevent skin from sagging.

113 UPLIFT WITH FIRMING TREATMENTS

Although there is little you can do to lift a sagging bosom apart from surgery, you can improve the skin texture and tone and temporarily firm the skin by using a serum specially formulated for this area. The skin will look less slack and appear tighter but the effect lasts only as long as you use the serum.

114 CHOOSE IDEBENONE

Look for skin-firming creams and serums specially formulated for the neck and décolletage areas, especially ones containing idebenone, a potent antioxidant that is claimed to alter the reaction of free radical damage and protect skin lipids. These creams are formulated to re-energize, firm, smooth and brighten the skin.

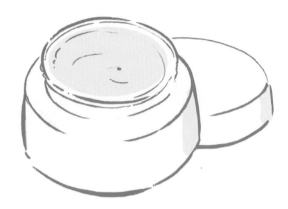

lips

117 LIP-PUMPING PEPTIDES

Products containing peptides that have been proven to boost collagen production may be your best shot for creating a soft, pillowy pair of lips without a needle in sight.

118 NO MORE ROUGH LIPS

Rough, unkissable lips should be treated with a natural exfoliating rub made from finely ground brown sugar and sesame oil. Scuff this delicious mixture gently over lips to remove dead and flaky skin. Finish with petroleum jelly.

119 MEND AN UNHAPPY MOUTH

Chapped lips that are dry, cracked and sore will look painful and interfere with many daily activities like eating – and kissing. To remedy the problem, use an oil-based chapstick or one that contains beeswax regularly, and avoid flavoured lip balms, as you will be tempted to lick them off and make the problem worse.

115 REMEMBER YOUR CLEAVAGE

When applying day or night cream, always remember to include your chest area from the top of your bust to your neck. Without extra moisturizer the skin here becomes thin and crêpe-like, and can be a telltale sign of ageing.

116 MINIMIZE NECK DAMAGE

Don't neglect to nourish your neck with a rich emollient night cream every evening before bedtime. The area from the collarbones up to the jawline often becomes prematurely wrinkled because the skin here is thinner and more vulnerable than that on your face.

120 RESCUE FLAKY LIPS

Try a two-step lip treatment to treat dry winter lips that are flaky and scaly. A lip exfoliator gently sloughs off dead and dull cells, before an intensive balm is applied to nourish and moisturize the new skin.

121 LIPS DON'T LIKE LICKING

When lips are exposed to harsh elements, we may be tempted to lick them to moisten the surface. This dries them out further because saliva contains enzymes that break down moisture, leaving them drier and thinner, which can add years to your look. Keep a small tin of shea butter in your bag and use it several times a day in winter.

hands & feet

122 KEEP HANDS HIDDEN

Wrinkled hands are the biggest telltale sign of ageing. Exposed to the elements nearly all the time, they take quite a battering, so cover them up and protect them wherever possible. Use rubber gloves to wash dishes, and gardening gloves when working outside.

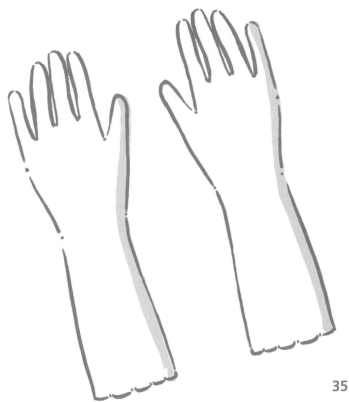

35

123 HANDS HATE WATER

The skin on the hands is thin and endlessly ravaged by the elements, so keep your hands dry as much as possible. Water left on the hands will evaporate, leaving them dried up and red. Use a hand cream that contains lanolin.

124 WAKE UP TO FABULOUS HANDS

Once a month cover your hands in thick nourishing cream, and slip them into soft cotton gloves for the night. In the morning all the cream will have been absorbed, leaving hands smoother and softer. It is also helpful to keep a regular supply of hand cream on the bedside table to remind you to apply it before you sleep.

125 OLD LADY HANDS

A salon-inspired handcare treatment that includes a self-heating exfoliant to skim off dry flaky skin, followed by a luxuriant hand cream to put back softness, will make a noticeable difference to wrinkled hands.

126 BE A BAREFOOT BEAUTY

For general foot health, try to reduce the amount of time you spend in shoes. At your work desk or at home, use every opportunity to slip off your footwear and walk around barefoot. This is particularly important if you are trying to prevent such conditions as bunions or calluses.

127 GOOD FOOT HEALTH

Nine out of ten women suffer from corns, calluses or bunions at some point in their life, and nine out of ten wear shoes that are too small. To prevent problems with your feet, ensure your shoes are the correct size and never wear the same ones two days in a row. Shoes that are too tight can eventually cause such debilitating conditions as hammertoes and bone spurs.

128 FEELING LIVERISH

Over-the-counter skin lighteners work by inhibiting the natural pigment called melanin, which lies deep in the skin, with an active ingredient called hydroquinone. It may take weeks for the new lightened skin cells to reach the surface and for the liver spots to reduce, but it does work.

129 HARSH CHEMICALS DAMAGE HANDS

Always wear rubber gloves when washing up dishes and rinsing through clothes. Unless your hands are protected, the harsh chemicals used in most washing-up liquids will leave your hands red and raw and very dehydrated.

130 GET A REGULAR PEDICURE

A professional pedicure can help address any foot care problems and also prevent future ones. In addition to a nail tidy, the treatment involves an exfoliation, a moisturizing treatment and an invigorating foot massage, to soothe rough and cracked skin.

131 CHOOSE MILD SOAP

If you wash your hands as often as you should during the course of 24 hours, make sure you are using a good-quality soap with natural ingredients like lemon or oatmeal. Cheap soaps leave hands dry and chapped.

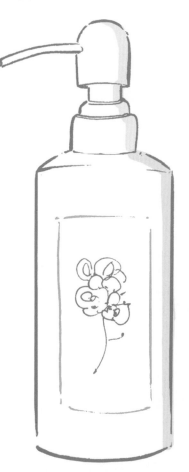

132 FOOT MASSAGE

A weekly home massage with a massage oil can not only help reduce any pain from years of accumulated stress on the feet, but it can soothe and hydrate rough skin and increase circulation to the extremities.

body treatments

133 HONEY HYDRATING WRAP

To rehydrate tired skin and replenish moisture, try a luxurious heated milk-and-honey body wrap at your favourite spa or salon. Honey acts as a natural humectant, and the warm treatment will leave aching muscles thoroughly relaxed.

134 ALWAYS REPLACE MOISTURE

Baths and showers always rob skin of its moisture, even if you use a very gentle body wash. Always use body oil or a specially formulated body lotion after bathing to replace lost moisture and keep skin hydrated.

135 LIGHTEN UP

Darker areas of skin, as at the knees and elbows, are the result of very dry skin and accumulated skin cells. These will benefit from an intensive exfoliation treatment, followed by a rich moisturizing cream. To lighten skin at the elbows, cut a lemon in half and rub each half into an elbow.

136 UPPER ARM FIRMER

The area directly above the outer elbow is one of the first places to show ageing saggy skin, yet it is often neglected because we never naturally see this part of our own body. It is also more resistant to the firming benefits of exercise than other parts, as there are no large muscle groups there. To help, try massaging a firming body or face cream into the area.

137 REJUVENATING BODY WRAP

Wrapping the body from chest to toes in a mineral-rich mud or seaweed-soaked cloth will invigorate tired skin, enhance circulation and help to detoxify, which will leave skin revitalized and glowing.

138 WAX YOUR KNEES AND ELBOWS

The skin at the knees and elbows is prone to sagging and dryness as there are few oil glands there. Ease rough, cracked skin with a paraffin treatment. Used medically to aid aching joints, warm nutrient-rich paraffin is brushed on the area and allowed to harden before being removed. The treatment aids circulation, softens rough skin, cleanses the pores and loosens the joints.

139 HOME SPA

To help keep it healthy and minimize the risk of illness, re-energize your body with a hydrotherapy bath. A warm bath can help revive joint and muscle pain, while a cold bath thins the blood, increases blood sugar and leaves the skin fresh and tingly.

140 THE WONDERS OF MESOTHERAPY

Mesotherapy involves the injection of vitamins, minerals and antioxidants into the middle layer of the skin. This is said to improve the quality and texture of the skin by replenishing essential vitamins that occur naturally within the cells.

141 FIRM UP FLABBY ARMS

Recognized as a fabulous treatment for cellulite, Velasmooth can work wonders on flabby arms. It involves three stages: infrared waves to boost the metabolic rate; radio frequency waves that shock and tighten the skin, causing it to lift and contract; and suction to pummel the skin and draw out toxins. Several treatments may be needed for long-lasting results.

142 FAT-BUSTING PLANTS

To stimulate the lymph flow and break down fatty tissue, natural plant extracts containing enzymes and nutrients can be injected into the middle layer of skin (mesoderm), using extremely small needles. A long-term course is recommended.

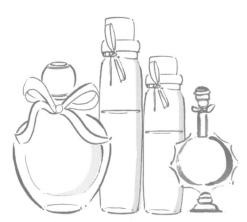

tackling cellulite

143 DETOX TO DUMP CELLULITE

Regardless of age, weight or body type, all women can suffer from cellulite. Getting rid of unwanted toxins and waste will allow your liver to metabolize fats more efficiently and reduce cellulite. Undertake a seven-day detox plan, combined with body brushing and massage, and you should see visible results.

144 CUT OUT CAFFEINE

Ingesting caffeine impairs circulation and lymph flow. Replace all caffeine drinks with detoxing green tea, dandelion tea or hot water with lemon and ginger.

145 RESHAPE WITH HYPOXITHERAPY

Eliminate fat and cellulite from the bottom and legs with a fat-burning treatment called Hypoxitherapy. Involving exercising and cycling under low atmospheric pressure, this increases blood supply and circulation and breaks down fatty deposits.

146 SKIN-FOLD MASSAGE

Endermologie was developed in France to reduce the appearance of cellulite. Focusing on areas that are prone to the problem like saddlebag thighs, bottoms and tummies, a suction-roller device smoothes the skin surface and stimulates the circulation by eliminating toxins in the tissues.

147 DAILY BODY BRUSHING

Get into the habit of body brushing every day to slough off dead skin cells, boost circulation and encourage new regeneration. Skin will look smoother as better circulation helps disperse fatty deposits.

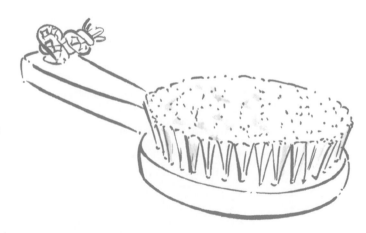

148 KNEAD AWAY LUMPS AND BUMPS

Vigorous massage will stimulate the circulation of the lymphatic drainage system and speed up toxin elimination. Target specific areas and simply massage in circular movements for a couple of minutes a day to help reduce cellulite, or have a professional lymphatic drainage massage.

149 SCRUB UP

A very hot bath, around 32°C (90°F), will open the pores and encourage the body to sweat, helping to release harmful toxins.

150 CIRCULAR BRUSHING STROKES

Using moderate pressure and short strokes with a natural bristle body brush, start brushing the skin in upward circular movement from the lower body up towards the heart. As well as stimulating blood circulation in the tiny capillaries near the skin, it will tone and tighten the skin and help reduce cellulite deposits.

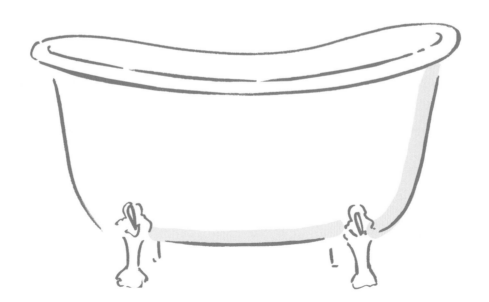

151 IMPROVE LEGS WITH BIRCH OIL

Combat ugly cellulite with regular massage. Diet and exercise are all known to help reduce the lumpy orange-peel skin that appears at the top of the thigh and on the bottom, but massage using a plant-based cream like birch oil helps too, by improving blood and lymph circulation, and releasing trapped toxins.

152 HAND MASSAGE FOR CELLULITE

Apply moisturizing cream to the area to be massaged and, using your thumb and forefingers, grip the skin and fatty layer beneath it and start to knead in small circular movements. Let your fingers glide smoothly over the skin and do not rub so hard that you bruise yourself.

153 TURN OFF THE HEAT

In the morning, jump-start your body by gradually turning your warm shower water to cold. Let it run for a minute all over your face and body to give the lymphatic system a boost, and tone up the skin to leave it tingling.

154 HIGH COLONIC CLEANSING

Constipation is one of the causes for toxins building up in your body and those toxins get trapped in connective tissue and appear as cellulite. Colonic cleansing, often used in conjunction with a detox, clears out the large intestine, killing harmful bacteria and parasites that live in the gut. A painless procedure performed by a therapist, it also helps the colon absorb vitamins, minerals and essential fatty acids more efficiently.

155 NATURAL SALT SCRUBS

For an invigorating body scrub, grab a handful of luxury salt granules, such as 'Fleur de Sel', and mix them with a tablespoon of good-quality almond oil. Massage gently over rough skin, paying particular attention to knees and elbows, then rinse off with warm water.

156 WRAP UP WARM

After a warm detox bath, wrap up warmly in thick layers of clothes and your body will continue to sweat out toxins for the next 30 minutes.

157 REDUCE WATER RETENTION

Water retention contributes to the appearance of cellulite, but don't choose commercial diuretics as they can leach potassium from the body, contributing to osteoporosis. Natural diuretics are dandelion, nettle, astragalus, juniper, parsley and vitamin B6, but the best method is to radically reduce your intake of salt and increase your intake of water.

158 HEALTHY LIFESTYLE

Although firming creams can help lumpy orange-peel skin to look firmer, they cannot penetrate deep into the dermal layers to change the skin's structure. For best results, ensure that you eat healthily and take adequate exercise.

159 SWEAT OUT TOXINS

Make your bathtime work for you by adding 450 kg (1 lb) of Epsom bath salts to the water. Epsom salts are made from the mineral magnesium sulfate, which draws toxins from the body, sedates the nervous system and relaxes tired muscles.

160 LASER LIGHT FIGHTS CELLULITE

Thought to temporarily reduce the appearance of cellulite, the Tri-Active laser combines suction massage to increase lymphatic drainage, which filters fluid from the cells. Low-intensity diodes heat to stimulate collagen production and tighten the skin, which is left visibly smoother.

161 BRAVE AN ICY DIP

Increase your metabolism by jumping into a freezing cold bath first thing in the morning. Within a few minutes, your blood and lymph circulation will increase, and the production of white blood cells will increase, destroying circulating toxins. Only do this if you are fit and healthy.

162 WRAP AWAY CELLULITE

Salon body wraps act on the principle of eliminating toxins and excess body fluids through sweating to reduce inches and improve the look of the skin. Used in conjunction with herbal preparations or creams, they have an immediate but temporary effect.

163 RIPPLES RESPOND TO TONING LIGHT

A successful Beverly Hills dermatologist has had good results on rippled cellulite using a device called the 'Galaxie', which is usually used for wrinkles. Radio frequency and laser light energy are directed beneath the skin's surface, to stimulate the production of new collagen and tighten the skin.

164 THREE MINUTES WITH A LOOFAH

Dry-brush your skin with a natural loofah first thing in the morning. You will feel the benefits as the accelerated blood flow invigorates you and sets your skin tingling – a great start to the day.

165 JUNK THE JUNK FOOD

Processed food contains artificial substances that the body finds hard to eliminate, and is a factor in the development of cellulite. Steer clear, too, of high GI foods like white bread, rice and potatoes that raise levels of fat-storing insulin. Stick to a diet that contains natural and organic meats and vegetables, which are simply cooked.

166 SWEAT IT OUT

Cleanse the body by spending half an hour in a steam room. The heat increases metabolism and pulse rate, and as blood vessels become more flexible, the whole body benefits from better circulation, leaving you feeling relaxed and energized – and all without moving a muscle.

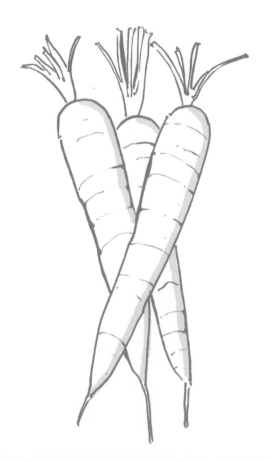

seasonal skincare

167 PERK UP WINTER SKIN

In extreme weather conditions cell renewal slows down, resulting in the skin thickening to protect itself and becoming less vibrant. To stop your skin becoming flat and grey, use super-hydrating serums packed with hyaluronic acid to nourish and remoisturize.

168 WISE UP TO WINTER

Harsh weather can lead to broken capillaries in the skin, caused by constant constricting and dilating of the blood vessels as you go from extreme cold outside to central heating inside. To support and strengthen capillary walls, increase your intake of vitamin C or use a serum containing high doses of vitamin C.

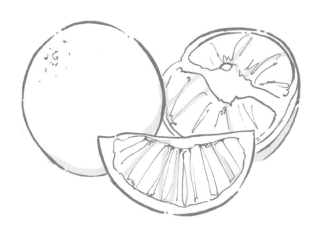

169 KEEP OUT OF THE WIND

Strong winds are harmful, as they cause moisture to evaporate, leaving skin dry, red and flaky. A skin cream that contains soy will form a protective barrier against the elements and give intense hydration to dry and itchy skin.

170 WATERPROOF YOUR SKIN

Older skin needs a protective barrier to guard against cold weather and moisture loss. Look for a humectant cream that provides environmental protection, and contains lipids and fatty acids to trap and retain moisture.

171 TURN OFF THE HEAT

Winter skin suffers from too much time spent indoors in a dry atmosphere. Healthy skin has a water content of between 10% and 20%, and central heating sucks natural moisture out, leaving skin dry and dull-looking. Lower the temperature of your heating, and increase your intake of water.

172 OVERNIGHT HYDRATION

During the night the skin rests and repairs itself after the stresses of the day. Use a humidifier or place a damp towel over your radiator at night to replace moisture in the air and keep the skin hydrated. This helps to humidify the air around you, and reduces excessive water loss from the skin.

173 EXTREME WEATHER FLUSH

Travelling between cold exteriors and warm interiors can create a flushed red-faced complexion, straining blood vessels in the skin, which change size rapidly as the temperature fluctuates. Find a cream that contains peptides to help plump up skin so the broken veins don't show.

174 TRY A TREATMENT MASK IN WINTER

Winter climates see a decline in the production of lipids (skin oils that seal in moisture). To compensate, try a revitalizing mask that contains a high amount of retinol, which stimulates elastin and collagen production, helping to plump up fine lines and even skin tone in more mature skin.

sun safety

175 PROTECT WITH PLE

If you are concerned about the effects of sun damage on the skin, consider taking an oral supplement that offers photo-protection, such as polypodium leucotomas extract, or PLE. Recent clinical research has found that this extract from a South American fern has powerful antioxidant and photoprotective properties. Native Americans have been using it to treat inflammatory disorders and skin diseases for centuries.

176 THE TAN WON'T LAST

As you age, the pigment in your skin becomes less active, with the result that your skin will tan less easily with time. Take notice of this simple fact to ensure that you don't accidentally stay out in the sun longer than is considered safe. If you like the look of a tan, rely on self-tanning products, which will be more effective than your own body's pigment-making capabilities.

177 A SAFE TAN

When our skin turns brown, it has been burnt, and damaged cells will always contain some residual changes that stay in our DNA and which may over time result in cancerous cells. The only safe tan is a fake one, where the active ingredient DHA reacts with proteins in our skin to stain it and make it darker in colour.

178 TAKE COVER AT THE HOTTEST TIME

Never spend more than four hours a day lying out in the sun, and take cover inside during the hottest hours of the day between 12 pm and 3 pm when the sun is at its most powerful and exposure of the skin should be avoided. Hair and eyes can also be damaged, so cover up with a broad-brimmed hat and sunglasses.

179 STAY YOUNG WITHOUT SUN

Exposure to sunlight leads to premature skin ageing and the cumulative effects of wrinkling, blotchy pigmentation and roughness. Sun-damaged skin is easier to bruise and is less elastic.

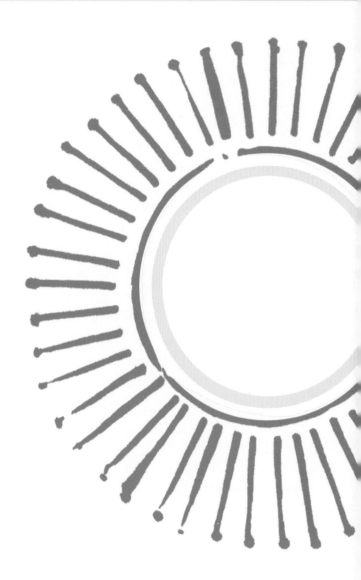

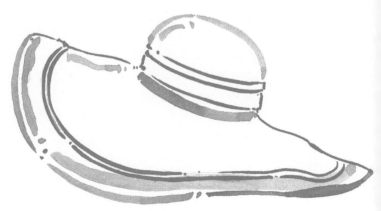

180 USE SPF 30 EVERY DAY

To avoid the damage the sun can do to your skin, it is essential to limit the time you expose your body to direct sunlight. You should always cover up your face with a sunscreen that has at least an SPF 30 and five-star UVA protection. Get into the habit of applying a sunscreen every day.

181 HANDS OFF

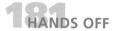

Sun damage affects all of your body, not just the face. Always remember to cover your hands with an SPF 20 when you spend time in the sun to avoid photo-ageing wrinkles and liver spots, the telltale signs of ageing.

182 SLAP IT ON

Most people apply suncream to their face and body at the start of the day and forget about it. During a typical two-week beach holiday, when you are exposed to the sun on a daily basis, you should expect to get through two 250 ml (8 fl oz) bottles of sun protection, so keep slapping it on all over throughout the day.

183 SHADES AND HAT COMPULSORY

Strong sunlight can damage the eyes, and particularly the fine skin around the eyes. Keep covered up throughout the day with sunglasses and a broad-brimmed hat to protect the face and hair.

184 DON'T DO SUNBEDS

Although a sunbed does not expose the body to UVB rays (the ones that affect the outer layers of the skin and cause sun damage), it can still cause burning and premature ageing because of the intensity of the UVA rays.

185 WINTER PROTECTION

Although we often remember to protect ourselves from the sun in summer, it is equally important throughout the year. Always wear a moisturizer with an SPF, and sunglasses when the winter sun appears, especially if you are out in the snow, which reflects the light.

186 CLOUDY DAY DAMAGE

Don't make the mistake of thinking your skin is safe from sun damage when the weather is overcast. Up to 80% of UV light can pass though cloud cover, so you still need protection on grey days and when sitting under a beach umbrella. Wear a daily moisturizer with SPF even when the sky is cloudy.

187 GLOBAL WARMING

If you want to avoid ageing liver spots and sun damage, you should be wearing an antioxidant moisturizer that contains a sunscreen all year round. Look for one that contains zinc oxide and titanium dioxide to block the sun.

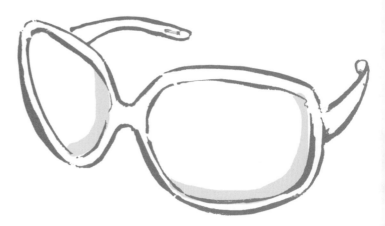

188 LEG CHECK

The most common place to develop a malignant melanoma is on your legs, so make sure you check them regularly for freckles or moles that have changed shape or are seeping blood. Don't be tempted to sunbathe without sun protection on your legs because you want to get them brown.

49

189 GET PREPARED

Don't wait until you are out in the sun to apply a protective lotion to your skin. Sunscreen needs time to work, so smooth it on about 20 minutes before you go outside, and don't be stingy with it – use liberal amounts.

190 DIFFERENT NEEDS

Your face and body require different products to protect them from sun damage. Always use SPF 30 on your face and at least an SPF 15 on your body, and make sure that your lotion has a high UVA filter.

191 SUN SAFETY FOR DARK SKINS

All skin needs protecting from harmful UVA and UVB rays, and while pale skin must use a higher SPF, even people with dark skin should never use anything lower than an SPF 15.

192 GREY DAY PROTECTION

A good day moisturizer not only kickstarts circulation after the nocturnal shutdown, but also helps to fight the damaging effects of the sun even in winter and on grey days.

193 GENETIC TESTING

A cancer expert has developed a new skin test called the Skinphysical, which can read the sun damage in your DNA. The results determine how much damage has already occurred and how to maximize your protection in future years. See www.skinphysical.co.uk.

194 SUN-SENSITIVE PERFUME

Avoid wearing fragrance that contains alcohol when sunbathing, as it makes skin photosensitive, and can result in dryness, burning and pigmentation. The eau de toilette version of your favourite perfume will usually have a lower alcohol content.

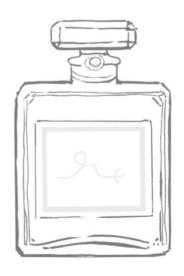

self-tanning

195 CHOOSE COLOURED SELF-TAN

The best self-tanners are those that are bronzed and instantly deposit a layer of non-permanent colour on the skin so you can see if you have missed any spots.

196 DON'T SWALLOW IT

The chemical DHA (dihydroxyacetone in spray-on tanners) is approved for external application only. Put cotton wool in your nostrils and keep your mouth closed during application in a tanning booth.

197 TAN FOR HEALTHY-LOOKING HANDS

Hands are one of the areas that show the most signs of ageing but they can look a lot better with a little light-coloured self-tan. This can be a tricky area to work on, so use your fingertips to lightly stroke and blend well, then use a facial wipe to clean the palms.

198 MAINTAINING THAT TAN

After a fake tan, use a light all-over body moisturizer to avoid flakiness. Take quick showers with minimal soaping (as opposed to luxurious bubble baths) and avoid heavy exercise, because sweat will dissipate the tan, leaving you covered in uneven patches.

199 PREP UP FOR GOOD TAN

A fake tan can even out the complexion and disguise dark circles and broken veins but won't work unless it's correctly applied. Thorough exfoliation of the skin is crucial for a good fake tan. Do it at home or get the therapist to do it before your treatment, followed by generous moisturizing to ensure colour goes on smoothly and there are no streaky stripes.

200 AIRBRUSH TAN IN A CAN

If you don't have the time (or money) for a trip to the salon, you can now buy a facial tanning spray in a can. With micro-fine particles you can expect to see professional results for a fraction of the cost, and not a patchy streak in sight.

condition
& care

201 HEALTH CHECK

Our skin and hair both reflect the overall state of our health, so if your hair looks dull and unhealthy, you need to check your nutritional intake. EFAs (essential fatty acids) are essential for glossy, vibrant hair, while zinc will help promote regrowth.

202 SUPER SHINE

For extra shiny hair, finish your final rinse with a blast of the most freezing cold water you can bear. It close the hair cuticles so that light bounces off them, resulting in super-shiny locks.

203 MAKE TIME FOR MASSAGE

When you apply conditioner, give yourself a slow fingertip scalp massage. Using gentle circular motions and a reasonable amount of pressure pushing down onto the scalp, you will boost blood circulation around the follicle and stimulate re-growth.

204 THE RIGHT SHAMPOO

If your hair has started to look dull, check the pH balance of your shampoo. The scalp's natural pH is between 4 and 6, but many shampoos are alkaline, which can make hair dull and unhealthy-looking.

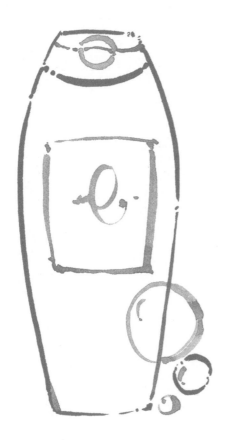

205 KEEP REGULAR APPOINTMENTS

Find a stylist you like and can trust to talk things through and discuss what is possible with your hair type and texture. Make regular appointments every 6–8 weeks for a trim, to keep your colour touched up and get an intensive conditioning treatment.

206 BE A HIGH-MAINTENANCE GIRL

As you get older, it is easier to cut corners on personal care and grooming – the other concerns of life can get in the way. But neglecting your hair can age you fast because it will look out of condition as well as out of style. Keep your standards high when it comes to looking after your hair – it needs your help more than ever as you age.

207 CONDITION WITH CARE

Some leave-in conditioners are unsuitable for fine hair. They coat the hair to protect it, but they can weigh it down and make it dull and greasy and very difficult to style. Wash-out conditioners generally suit all hair types better.

208 DON'T SKIMP ON CONDITIONER

Most hairdressers agree that healthy hair cannot be acquired from a bottle but that even if you skimp on the less expensive brands of shampoo, it is always worth investing in a good-quality conditioner. It is the equivalent of a face cream for your hair.

209 SPLASH OUT ON GOOD PRODUCTS

Many supermarket shampoos and conditioners contain very cheap ingredients, like ammonium laurel sulfate, which are harsh on your hair. Buy good-quality salon products and you will notice the difference in shine and texture.

210 HAIR ANALYSIS EATING STRATEGY

Mineral-testing a small lock of hair can reveal your metabolic type, toxin levels, health status and nutritional imbalances. Analyzing the biochemical make-up of an individual, and taking remedial action, can result in clearer skin, shinier hair, increased energy and even weight loss.

211 BEAUTY AND THE BEAST

Bull's semen is the latest hair care treatment used to provide pure protein for dry, coarse hair. The intense conditioner, which also contains the root of the protein-rich plant katera, is massaged into the hair, which is then treated with a steamer. This allows the product to penetrate deep into the hair before it is washed off, leaving soft and shiny locks.

212 CHECK LABELS FOR ALCOHOL

Some hair products contain alcohol, which can make hair drier than normal. If hair is coloured, it tends to make it dull and less vibrant. So look carefully at the list of ingredients and avoid this ingredient.

213 SMOKING DAMAGES YOUR HAIR

Smoking is very damaging, as it affects the take-up of vitamin C and constricts the blood vessels. This means that fewer nutrients needed for hair growth are getting through. Stop smoking and you will see instant results.

214 ADD MOISTURE WITH A MASK

If you feel your hair needs a pick-me-up, try using an intensive conditioner or hair mask that can be left on for 10 minutes to moisturize the hair shafts. While you are waiting, wrap your hair up in a warm towel to enable the treatment to penetrate more deeply.

215 NATURALLY STRONGER

If your hair has become weaker and more brittle, and has a tendency to break easily, try an infusion of rosemary poured over as a final rinse to strengthen it. Alternatively, massage some rosemary essential oil (mixed with a carrier oil) into your scalp to help promote growth and strength.

216 SHINE WITH SILICA

Studies have shown that this vital mineral can stimulate healthier hair growth, and make hair stronger as well as shinier. It is found in red and green peppers, or it can be taken as a supplement.

217 EAT NUTS FOR HEALTHY HAIR

Calcium, magnesium and potassium are all essential for the growth of thick, healthy hair. Snack regularly on almonds that are packed with these nutrients and contain more calcium than any other nut.

218 HOT HONEY HAIR

Give your hair and scalp a treat with an organic honey and olive oil conditioner. Mix equal parts together and warm in the microwave, then apply to clean, towel-dried hair, and wrap in a warm towel for 20 minutes. This will leave hair smooth and ultra-soft and shiny.

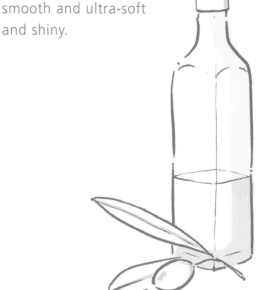

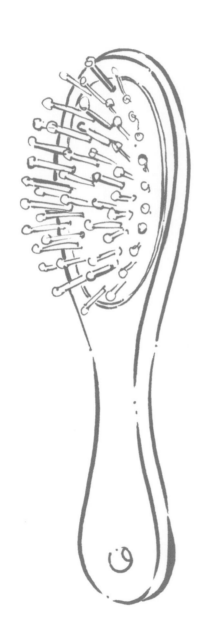

219 LEAVE IT LOOSE IN BED

Never jump into bed with your hair tied up in a scrunchy, or with clips and pins still in it. Your movements throughout the course of the night will damage and break your hair as it rubs against the pillows.

220 ONE HUNDRED OF THE BEST

Don't use a brush on wet hair, as this could damage it. Instead, use a wide-toothed comb to gently ease out knots. But giving dry hair the traditional brushing before bedtime will benefit your locks because it stimulates growth and oil production. Natural bristle brushes are gentlest on the hair.

221 GREAT LENGTHS

Hair products containing copper peptides have already shown a remarkable ability to increase growth. The mineral is thought to increase thickness and reduce brittleness in hair.

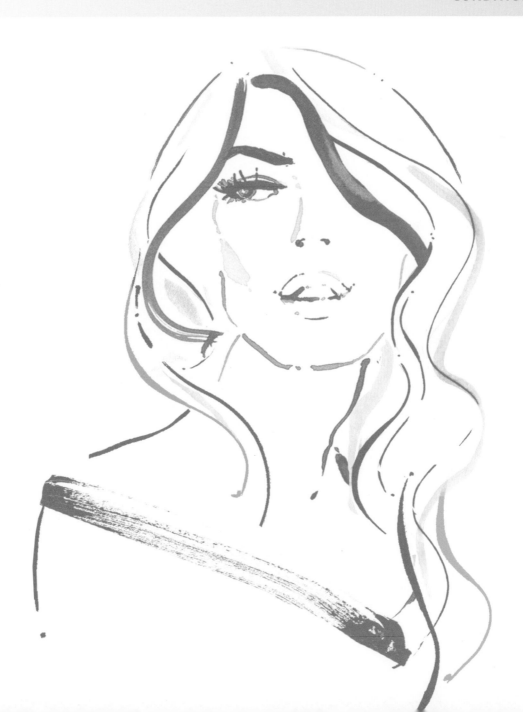

cuts & lengths

222 A PROFESSIONAL CUT

A good hair cut can take years off your perceived age and give you buckets of self-confidence. Regardless of your age, your hair should look soft and flattering, and a clever cut will emphasize all your good points while drawing attention away from your bad ones.

223 GET THE BEST FROM YOUR STYLIST

Book a quiet appointment time, like first thing on a Monday morning. When the salon is quiet, your hairdresser will have more time to focus on you, and give you exactly what you want.

224 READ A MAGAZINE

Take a look at some of the hair magazines on offer, as they will be showing the season's latest styles, cuts and colours. Even if they seem a little young or trendy to you, there are often ways of adapting them that can keep you in fashion but also within your comfort zone.

225 CALL A FRIEND

Ask a friend or family member for their opinion but be prepared that they might not be flattering. An honest opinion delivered by someone who knows you can really put you in touch with what's not working for you. Remember that they are probably more used to your face and the way it looks in various situations than you are.

226 ALL CHANGE

It's important to keep 'tweaking' your hairstyle and not to become trapped in a style that suited you when you were a teenager. Sometimes the best way to change your style is to try a new stylist or go to a salon that has a different approach from your usual one. All it takes is for someone to see you in a slightly new way.

227 DON'T GO TOO SHORT

Unless you have an amazingly elfin face, short cropped hair can look very butch and severe. Try a short bob instead, which is sleek and sophisticated and suits a greater variety of face shapes.

228 INDULGE IN A LITTLE CHIT-CHAT

Always find time for a five-minute chat with your hairdresser to discuss exactly what you want. This time is vital for them to look at the texture of your hair and your face shape before they start to work on you. If you've been with them for a while, they will also be able to pick up on changes that you might not have noticed – such as a few more grey hairs, thinning, or poor condition or split ends – and find remedies for them.

229 DON'T GO TOO LONG

Very long hair, way down your back, can look far too teenage once you are past 35; in fact, it can make you look a lot older than you are. If you love your long hair and don't want to give it up, try trimming off just 5 cm (2 inches) and seeing what it looks like. If you like it, get a little more trimmed off. You may find your face becomes the focal point rather than your hair, with a prettier result!

230 FLATTERING CUTS

Make your haircut work for you. Choose a hairstyle that has a side fringe (bangs) rather than a straight-across fringe, and a length that falls to just below the chin if you want to cover a wrinkled forehead and sagging jaw.

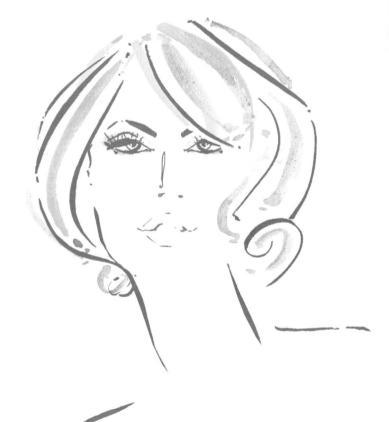

231 THE PERFECT LENGTH

The most flattering and youthful hair length, post 40, is to just below the chin to cover the jawline. This length works on nearly all women, and the hair can swing above the shoulder.

232 HEAVY HAIR SHADOWS SKIN

A thick and solid curtain of glossy hair can overwhelm the face and make skin look dull and tired. Shorter layers, cut through from underneath, are needed to give movement around the face and let light shine through.

233 DON'T TRY THIS AT HOME

Good grooming is essential as you get older, so make sure you invest in regular salon visits. If you used to cut your own hair in your twenties, don't even think about doing it now. Resist the urge to just trim your fringe (bangs) when it gets longer, too; many salons offer a free fringe trim between sessions, as this is the first area to grow out.

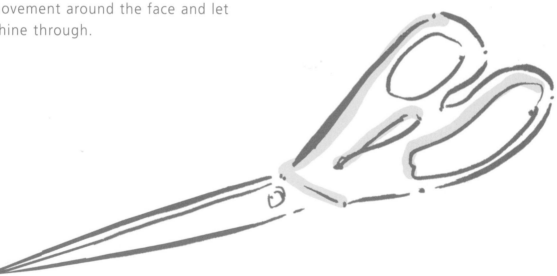

234 A LONG BOB

If your hair is in good condition and you are prepared to spend time blow-drying, a long bob is a good option, as the hair swings to create movement and will cover a jowly jawline and wrinkled neck.

235 AN UNFORGIVING CUT

Cropped hair can look fabulous on older women, but avoid a close-cut crop if you are bigger than a size 14 (US size 10), as visually it does not balance a larger frame.

236 A FEATHER CUT

If you want to disguise, or draw attention away from, crow's-feet, try a feathered cut or one that falls naturally forwards around the side. Avoid scraping your hair back off your face.

237 WITH A FRINGE ON TOP

A badly wrinkled forehead is easy to cover up with a fringe (bangs). Depending on your face shape, your fringe can be straight and solid or soft and wispy, but it will do the trick of hiding frown lines.

238 KEEP HAIR SOFT

Blunt geometric bobs that need a blast of hairspray to keep them in place can look hard and severe as the face ages and loses its youthful bloom. A good haircut for an older woman needs to have movement and softness around the face.

239 CUTS THAT FLATTER

Try to avoid having layered short cuts because they can be very ageing as they expose a saggy, wrinkled neck. If you have your hair a little longer, consider just feathering the fringe (bangs) and sides, which will keep the look soft and flattering.

240 AGE-APPROPRIATE HAIR

As you age, your hair thins and becomes much more wiry to the touch. Stay clear of the long, flowing locks you had when you were 18: your hair no longer has any of the same characteristics that made the style work back then.

thinning hair

241 EXTEND YOUR LOCKS

As age takes its toll on the speed of hair growth, you can always cheat a little with some longer extensions. The process is lengthy, and extensions need to be put in professionally, but they can add volume and length very successfully. If your hair is very thin, keep them at shoulder-length or above.

242 KNOW THIN FROM FINE

Thin hair and fine hair are different and need to be treated differently. Thin or 'low-density' hair has a less-than-average number of strands per square centimetre, so that the scalp can sometimes be seen through the hair. This can be in patches or all over. Fine hair, which you can have in abundance, refers to the thickness of the strands and can resemble thin hair because both types tend to be flat and lie close to the head.

243 ADD VOLUME WITH LAYERS

Choose a style that falls above the shoulder line, and that has layers cut into it for extra volume. Always use volumizing shampoos and styling products. A little mousse can be used to pump up the layers, but be careful not to overload the hair with product.

244 USE VOLUMIZING SHAMPOO SPARINGLY

Avoid using a specially formulated volumizing shampoo all the time, because the proteins they use to bond with the hair can build up as a residue and make hair look dull and lifeless.

245 SEAWEED REMEDY

To improve the thickness and condition of your hair, take a daily sea kelp supplement. This broad-fronded seaweed comes in several varieties but all are rich in potassium, calcium, magnesium and iron.

246 THIN HAIR SOLUTIONS

If you find your hair losing body as well as volume as you age, you need to find a style that incorporates some layering, whatever the length. Keeping hair cut all the same length can drag it down and make it look even thinner.

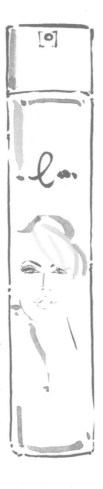

247 THIN ON TOP

Hair naturally thins out as part of the ageing process, as the number of follicles capable of growing hairs gradually declines. A straight parting with hair that just hangs down from it on either side will emphasize the problem, so ask your stylist to create a style that incorporates colour and texture.

248 FINE-HAIR FULLNESS

Traditional layers do not work as well for fine hair unless they are simple bevelled edges. Instead, try a perm, which thickens the diameter of the strands. This can be done on large rollers, to create waves rather than the classic kinky perm you might remember from your youth.

249 COLOUR-CORRECT THIN HAIR

Avoid all-over flat colour and try several shades of high- and lowlights instead. These add body and contrast to the hair, creating the illusion of depth.

250 VOLUMIZE THIN HAIR

After washing your hair, apply a thickening spray and blow-dry through, using your fingers to create a messy, tousled look. This look works best on mid-length layered cuts.

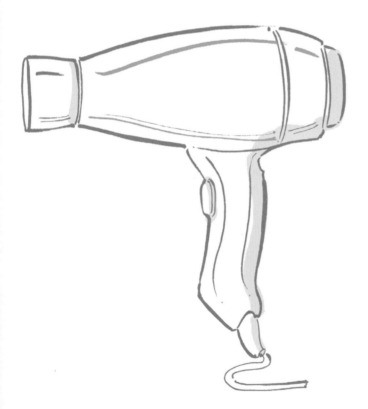

251 GUARD AGAINST HAIR LOSS

Thinning hair that falls out in clumps can come about as a result of a restricted diet. Hair loss from a lack of vitamins B and C and iron can be rectified with a diet rich in protein and vegetables. Packed with EFAs (essential fatty acids), flax seeds will make hair thicker and shinier.

252 PREVENTION IS THE BEST CURE

Breakages and poor condition are some of the reasons hair thins, so take steps to prevent hair loss by restricting the use of blow-dryers – extreme heat can break down the proteins in hair – straighteners or chemical treatments such as perms, straightening agents and colouring. The more you abuse your hair, the more risk there is of long-term damage.

253 CLEVER COVER-UP

If you find your hair thinning at your parting line, pull the front section of hair up over the top of your head and secure it with a clip at the crown, to cover up the parting.

254 AVOID TIGHT STYLES

Tight ponytails or cornrows can put stress on hair and increase the chance of breakages and hair loss. Frequently winding the hair around rollers, particularly the non-foam varieties, can also worsen hair loss.

255 USE VOLUMIZING SHAMPOO SPARINGLY

Avoid using a specially formulated volumizing shampoo all the time, because the proteins they use to bond with the hair can build up as a residue, which will make hair look dull and lifeless.

256 GET WIGGY WITH IT

If ageing has caused your hair to thin down so much that you can see your scalp through it, then a good-quality wig is an option. Get it cut and thinned down to the right weight for you by a professional hairdresser.

weather conditions

257 SUNLIGHT STEALS MOISTURE

A summer holiday will leave your hair feeling dry and brittle, as the UV rays suck out moisture. Every other day on holiday, try a leave-in conditioner that has a UV filter for protection.

258 SUNSHINE INCREASES THE GREASE

Hot summer sunshine can increase sweat production and make your scalp look and feel much greasier. To counteract this problem, try more frequent washing with a small amount of shampoo, and use a much lighter conditioner.

259 DETOX POLLUTED HAIR

In the summer months, there are higher levels of humidity and pollution in the air, so hair should be washed and conditioned more frequently using a good detox shampoo, which will clean the hair gently without stripping away natural oils.

260 SUNLIGHT DAMAGES PRODUCTS

Keep conditioners and styling products away from the beach, as they need to be stored in a cool, shady place. Exposure to strong sunlight will destroy some of the active ingredients that make these hair products work.

261 REMEDY SCARECROW HAIR

A week of sun, salt water and chlorine will all play havoc with your hair, so spend one day with your hair covered in an intensive conditioner, slicked back and covered with a fashionable Pucci- or Hermes-style scarf. This eight-hour treatment will restore your hair to its pre-holiday condition.

262 WIND WARNING

In summer, a combination of strong winds on a sandy beach can cause as much damage as the sun, so occasionally use a good 'leave-in conditioner' on your hair for the day. Choose one that contains Vitamin B5, which will nourish and protect your hair from beach damage.

going grey

263 GREY HEADS GO BLONDE

Occasionally grey hair can acquire a yellow tint; this can be avoided by choosing shampoos and conditioners that have been specially formulated for highlighted hair.

264 FADE TO GREY

When our bodies stop producing the pigment melanin, our hair starts to turn grey. This won't happen overnight, but having highlights around the crown will soothe the transition to a full head of grey hair, and will help create warmth and depth to the salt-and-pepper colour, whatever your style.

265 GREY MATTERS

By the age of 50, 50% of women will be 50% grey. Grey hair doesn't have to mean 'old' hair. No matter what the shade, hair is an extension of who we are, and if it is glossy, well cared for and cut regularly, you will look fabulous whatever your colour.

266 A BRAND NEW SHADE

If you find yourself with too much grey hair and want to turn back the clock to how it used to look, never go for the exact same shade; try one shade lighter, as it will be more flattering to your skin tone.

267 THE HIGHS AND LOWS

As the number of grey flecks in your hair start to increase, highlighted hair becomes less flattering. Try asking for highlights and lowlights at the same time to complement your new salt-and-pepper growth.

268 FIRST GREY HAIRS

At the beginning of the greying process, usually around your late thirties, follicles produce colourless strands in a random pattern, often on the temples and the top of your head. Darker hairs normally hide the grey strands when they first appear. At this stage it is unlikely that anyone other than you will notice the grey. If you are worried, changing your parting may make those strands a little less noticeable.

269 AVOID SMOKING TO STOP GREY

The age at which you start to go grey and by how much is largely a matter of genetics, but there are other contributing factors. A 1996 *British Medical Journal* study reported that smokers are four times more likely to go grey at a young age.

270 WHITEN THE GREY

Technically there is no such hair colour as grey. Hair is either pigmented or it is white – the grey is simply a mixture of white hair and coloured hair. If your grey hair looks dull, consider using a silver shampoo formula, which will brighten both the white and pigmented strands and give them lustre.

271 HAIR LOSS MAKES GREY MORE OBVIOUS

Drug treatments for illnesses, even if they are alternative medicine, can arrest the growth cycle of hair and cause it to fall out, as can alopecia, a condition that causes hair loss. When hair is lost, more of the existing greys may be revealed.

272 FEED YOUR HAIR

Because hair grows with the melanin pigment inside, no external cause will make you go grey. To help keep melanin production at the highest possible level, ensure you are getting enough of the mineral copper in your diet. Food that contains good supplies includes crab, oysters, sunflower seeds and nuts.

273 WHEN TO COVER THE GREY

If your hair is just beginning to change colour, with the grey making up less than 20% of it, use a semi-permanent colour that will begin to fade in about 6–12 washes. For up to 50% grey, opt for a semi-permanent that is claimed to last for about 24 washes. Only choose a permanent dye if the majority of your hair has turned grey. If you're mostly grey, consider a shade slightly darker than your normal colour, because the colour may fade with exposure to sun and shampooing.

274 RESTRICT YOUR DIET

To prevent premature greying some nutritionists recommend restricting your intake of caffeine, alcohol, meat and any food that is fried, greasy, spicy, sour or acidic. These items are said to reduce moisture and nutrients from reaching the hair follicles.

colours & highlights

275 GO SLOWLY WITH COLOUR

When changing your colour, go slowly and naturally, starting with highlights and/or lowlights rather than opting for a full colour change immediately. You do not want your hair to look out-of-sync with your age – very dark or very blonde hair will immediately look artificial on anyone over the age of 30. Your hair colour should keep up with the changes in your skin condition and tone – that way, it will look more natural.

276 DON'T DIY

Resorting to products from the chemist may end in disaster and ultimately you will have to visit a salon to put everything right, at greater expense than if you had gone there in the first place. Never correct your colour by yourself, as it will only compound the problem, but visit a salon and get professional advice.

277 LIGHTEN UP

As skin loses melanin and becomes paler in colour, think about changing your hair colour to complement your skin. Adding darker shades will drain the colour from your face, whereas a mixture of lighter shades with darker tones underneath will create texture and movement.

278 FRINGE BENEFITS

All types of fringes (bangs) can be flattering to older faces, but they should never look neglected with root regrowth. Most salons offer special fringe colouring services, so keep yours fully highlighted, to lift the look of your face and the rest of your hair.

279 AVOID EXTREME COLOUR

Peroxide blonde and Cruella de Ville black are both very difficult shades to wear successfully as you get older. These extreme shades will draw attention to the face, and you will need superb make-up at all times to balance the effect of such dramatic hair.

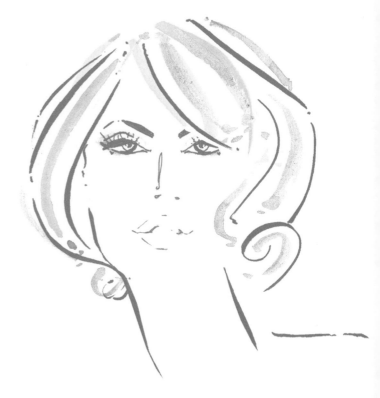

280 HIGHLIGHT HOLIDAY HAIR

Hair that has been over-bleached is most susceptible to the ravages of sun, sea and chlorine damage. To minimize damage, just get your parting highlighted before a holiday. It's a cheaper option and will save you from chemical overload.

281 BEWARE THE BOTTLE BLONDE

If you want to warm up your blonde hair, choose some natural shades of high- and lowlights, as bright flat peroxide blonde is very ageing. Know the correct blonde for your skin tone – if you have a 'cool' skin tone, choose ash, mink and platinum shades, not warm golds or coppers, which are better for warm complexions.

282 KEEP IT UNDER WRAPS

Maintain colour-treated hair by keeping it from undue exposure to sunlight and chlorine. Use a bathing cap when you swim, wear hats in very sunny or poor weather and use a good-quality shampoo, formulated to help resist colour fade.

283 CHECK OUT YOUR BROWS

Often the colour of the eyebrows fades as you get older and you will need to assess your hair colour in conjunction with them. If you don't, you run the risk of having a beautiful head of hair that is let down by pale or greying brows. Get the objective professional advice of a colourist before making any colour decisions.

284 COLOUR ME BEAUTIFUL

Changing hair colour to warm up a mousy brown or cover the odd streak of grey can take years off your age. For the most natural look, it's best to stay within two or three shades of your original colour, and always consider your skin tone.

285 BEWARE SUN-IN PRODUCTS

Never use sun-lightening products such as lemon juice or over-the-counter products that are meant to lighten hair in the sun, or you may soon find yourself needing a short haircut to prune away the damage.

286 LAY OFF THE HENNA

If your own colour now contains more than 50% white, you should avoid henna treatments, as they will appear very bright orange.

287 SUN-KISSED MOUSY BLONDES

As you age, the skin gets paler and loses colour, so mousy hair should be lifted with warm golden highlights to add warmth to your face. Adding darker shades will drain even more colour from your skin.

288 DULL HIGHLIGHTS

In between trips to the salon, perk up dull highlights by using a colour-enhancing treatment, or adding vitamin E oil capsules to your weekly hair mask, to brighten colour and add shine.

289 COVER UP COLOUR TREATMENTS

Keep coloured hair under a scarf or broad-brimmed hat when you are out in the sunshine. UVA rays will lift the colour, and leave you rushing to the hairdresser.

290 SHOP AROUND

There are so many different types of products available for every different type of hair, so make sure you find the right formula for you. Coloured hair needs a colour-formulated shampoo that will cleanse gently and not strip the colour out.

291 CUT DOWN ON CHEMICALS

Professional hairdressers suggest that in order to keep hair as healthy as it can be, you choose only one chemical treatment at a time. For example, perming and colouring together will leave hair weak, chemically damaged and very brittle.

292 HOLIDAY HAIR CARE

Always wash your hair as soon as possible after swimming in the sea or a chlorinated swimming pool. Coloured and treated hair are prone to damage and fading if sea salt or chemicals are left in the hair, especially if you intend to spend time out in the sun after your swim.

293 KEEP A REGULAR TOUCH-UP

Nothing is more ageing than large grey roots on coloured hair. In order to avoid this, you will have to make sure you book an appointment at least every six weeks.

294 GO FOR RED

An alternative to natural highlights and lowlights is a whole head colour change to either soft red or burnt copper, both of which are good choices for older skin tones.

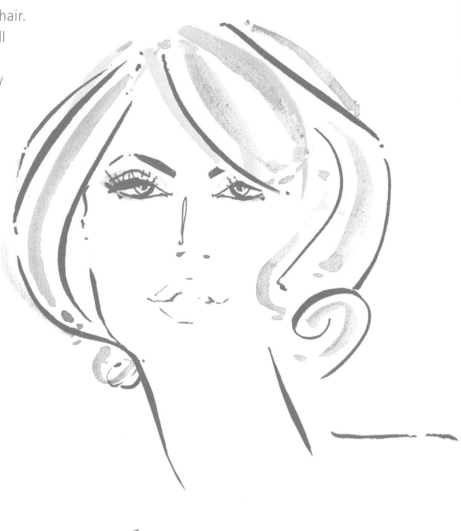

styling secrets

295 PICK AND CHOOSE PRODUCTS

Choose the right products for your hair type, which will change throughout your life, depending on environmental factors, stress and dietary changes. If you have oily roots and dry ends, find a shampoo for oily hair and concentrate on lathering at the roots: the rest of your hair will still get clean.

296 OVER-BRUSHING CAN BE DAMAGING

Always use a good-quality brush to style your hair but do not over-brush it, as with every stroke you will damage your hair more and create more split ends.

297 COMB, DON'T BRUSH

When hair is damp or wet, it is much weaker and more easily damaged. Always treat wet hair carefully and use a wide-toothed comb to straighten out tangles, and never a brush, which will create split ends.

298 DON'T OVERDO THE STRAIGHTENING IRONS

If you want to straighten your hair on a daily basis, alternate your use of straightening irons with a hand-held dryer. With a dryer, the heat comes from just one source and is not so damaging for your hair, leaving it less dry and in better condition.

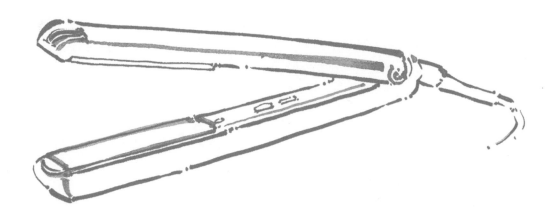

299 INSTANT LIFT AND BOUNCE

For a quick fix of volume, spray a small amount of thickener or volumizer onto the pieces of hair at the front of your face. Roll up on big Velcro rollers, and blast with a burst of hot air from a dryer. Undo gently for instant lift.

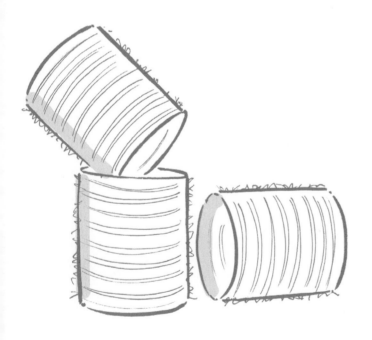

300 LAY OFF THE HEAT

Long-term use of heated appliances will damage your hair by drying out the shaft. If you avoid using heated products every day of the week and save them for special occasions, you will start to notice the improvement in the texture of your hair within weeks.

301 MAKE A BIG IMPRESSION

Root-lift without a salon blow-dry can be achieved by a quick 10-minute upside-down root blast with a professional high-watt hairdryer. There's no need to wash your hair first, as it works better on slightly dirty hair, giving immediate lift and body.

302 CHECK OUT STYLING PRODUCTS

Hair changes as you get older, and you may need to consider products you have never used before. These can add volume, give root-lift, add gloss, help control static and protect the shaft from heated styling appliances. Check them out to make the most of your hair.

303 SALON SMOOTHIE

For salon-styled hair, always divide your hair into manageable sections. The more you do, the better the result. Point the hairdryer downwards to close hair shafts, making hair look ultra-sleek.

304 AVOID CUTESY ACCESSORIES

Pigtails and bunches are best left to 10-year-olds. Plastic bobbles, floral clips and glitter scrunchies will only serve to emphasize your lack of youthfulness.

305 HOT HAIR NEEDS HOT AIR

If you want to re-create salon-styled hair, you will need a dryer with a nozzle to diffuse the heat. Hold the dryer as far as possible away from the hair and keep it moving around to minimize damage to the hair shafts.

306 BACKCOMB TO BUILD UP

If your hair has lost some of its natural body, a quick way to add volume without blow-drying is to backcomb very gently with a wide-toothed comb, and then spray with a light-formula superfine setting mist.

307 SIMPLE AND STYLISH

A style that incorporates lots of hair clips or decorations is best reserved for the under-30s. Zany, oddball or cute isn't the look to cultivate – instead think sexy, stylish and chic. Erring on the side of simplicity, with a great cut and colour, will make heads turn for all the right reasons.

308 BAD HAIR DAYS

Studies at Yale University show that 'bad hair days' really can effect self esteem, increase self-doubt and intensify insecurities. Women perceive their capabilities to be significantly lower when their hair doesn't look good, so time spent with the dryer is time well spent.

309 BLOT UP EXCESS MOISTURE

Between showering and drying your hair, always blot hair dry with a fresh towel to absorb excess water. If you then apply a heat-activated product that coats and protects the hair shaft, you will minimize damage from the hairdryer and keep your hair in optimum condition.

310 STYLE IT QUICKLY

After showering, wrap hair gently in a towel, choose and apply the correct amount of styling product and then blow-dry. Damp hair that is moisture-laden will help styling products work better, and you will achieve better results.

311 EXTRA SHINE

If you want to make straight hair even glossier, blow-dry in the usual way and then brush through for 5 minutes from root to tip with a paddled shaped hairbrush with good-quality bristles.

312 LOOK AT THE OVERALL PICTURE

Some women look great with trendy, spiky, short styles and can wear them into their seventies with great aplomb, whereas others in their twenties wouldn't be able to carry the look off. The key is to consider not only the quality and texture of your hair but also your bone structure, as well as your build, personality and dress sense. For a look to work well, all these factors need to be in tune.

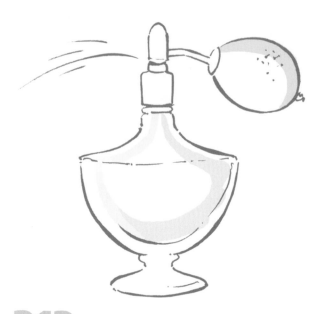

313 SWEET-SMELLING HAIR

Before you go out, spritz fragrance through your hair, which is more porous than skin, so you will retain the sweet-smelling aroma for longer.

314 POWER DRY

For a professional finish at home, look for a good-quality dryer that has between 1200 and 2000 watts. When you use it, keep the heat setting on low and the dryer moving around so that heat damage is kept to a minimum.

315 WEAR A HAT

If your roots are showing a little too much or your hair is lifeless and flat – or you simply haven't had time to look after it properly – solve the problem by donning a stylish hat. If you hate hats, try a stylish scarf or hair band to keep your locks under control.

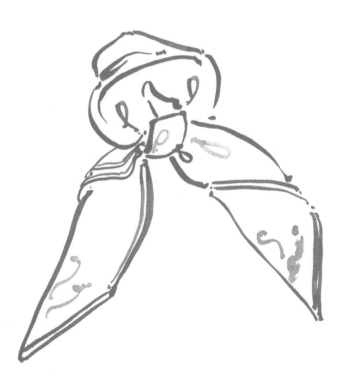

316 LET YOUR HAIR DOWN

If you have a slack jawline, avoid putting your hair up in a bun or chignon. No matter how sleek-looking, these are looks that are best suited for those with perfect profiles. Such styles can also make a thin face look even thinner – having some volume around the chin creates a more youthful fullness and hides the jawline at the same time.

317 LESS IS MORE

Don't overdo the styling products or the amount of product you use. You won't get a better result by squirting a huge amount of mousse onto your hair; most professionals recommend a golf ball-size blob of mousse. Otherwise hair can end up looking sticky and flat.

318 EXPERIMENT AT HOME

Even something as simple as changing your parting line can make you look younger. Take a pile of magazine cuttings, a comb and some clips, and experiment in front of the mirror to try out different styles.

319 TRY IT ON FIRST

If you are thinking about making some radical changes to your hair, it's worth doing a little experimenting first. Try on different wigs to get some idea of how you might look with a new cut or colour. If you fancy hair extensions, have a play with some at-home clip-on extensions first before splashing out on the more expensive salon versions.

320 BAND AID

Tying a tight black hairband up over the forehead will keep your hair sleek and tidy and help keep wrinkles pulled back. Backcomb hair slightly and let it fall down over the band like a sexy 1950s film star.

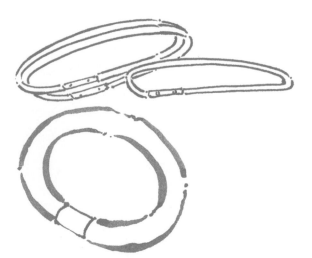

321 PONYTAIL PULL-UP

Try wearing your hair up in a high, sleek ponytail. It pulls the skin up towards the crown, making it appear taut and smooth, and looks tidy and chic.

troubleshooting

322 TEA TREATMENT

Greasy hair will benefit from a weekly treatment of cold peppermint tea, poured over the hair after washing. It will also make your hair smell fresh and minty for 24 hours.

323 STRESS-RELATED DANDRUFF

Internal stress and conflict trigger many physical signs that your life is unbalanced. When the glands that produce oil start overworking, dead cells fall off in clumps rather than one by one, and cause dandruff. Try using a shampoo containing zinc, sulphur or selenium.

324 FLAKY WHITE DANDRUFF

The shiny white scales that separate from the scalp and collect on the hair and shoulders are almost always caused by impaired general health. Increase your intake of raw foods that are high in enzymes (fruit, vegetables and nuts) and take two dessertspoons of flax oil a day until the condition improves.

325 REPAIR CENTRAL-HEATING DAMAGE

The contrast of chilly outdoor temperatures and warm central heating can cause a dry, itchy scalp. Look for a mild shampoo from an organic range, which will be kind to your hair and provide it with plant-based extractions to soothe the scalp.

326 KITCHEN COLOUR CORRECTOR

If blonde hair turns a strange shade of 'green' after a summer spent swimming in chlorinated pools, comb tomato ketchup through and leave for 20 minutes. Then, wash and condition in the usual way.

327 EMERGENCY HAND CREAM FOR HAIR

In an emergency you can use a tiny amount of light hand cream to control frizzy hair without damaging it. Rub a small amount of cream into your hands, and when it is almost absorbed, run your hands very lightly down the length of your hair. Make sure you give your hair a deep conditioning treatment the next day.

328 MOISTURIZE YOUR SCALP

A flaky scalp can be a sign of dryness and a result of poor diet, stress or fluctuating hormones. It should be treated with products that add moisture like aloe-vera shampoo and conditioner.

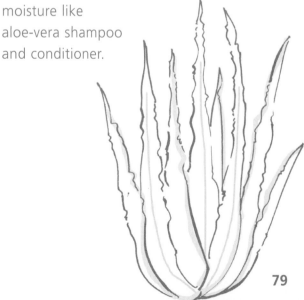

79

antiageing make-up tips

329 GET OUT OF THE RUT

If you wear the same style of make-up that you did when you were in school, it's time to make some changes. Visit your favourite make-up counter and ask a professional make-up artist to show you how to enhance your best features.

330 MAGNIFY YOUR MAKE-UP

If you can't see without your glasses, consider buying a pair of special make-up glasses to help you put your eye make-up on. The lens can be moved from either side of the frame, so one side of the face can be made up using magnification, and then changed over.

331 DITCH THE JUNK

Throw away your old broken compacts and dried-up tubes of lipgloss on a regular basis, and look for multiple-use products that will reduce the need to carry so much junk around with you.

332 CONSULT A CONSULTANT

Make-up products are changing rapidly, and for the better. If you are confused by too much choice and don't know your 'concealer' from your 'corrector', book an appointment at the counter of your favourite brand and ask for advice on new products and how to apply them.

333 CHOOSE DAYLIGHT TO MAKE UP

Always apply daytime make-up using daylight, as your skin will change with the season. Set up a magnifying mirror near a window with a good source of natural light, and make sure shading is properly blended for the most natural-looking face.

334 CHANGE DIRECTION

Change the tools you use to apply your make-up. Buy a set of different-sized brushes, powder puffs and sponges, and use a new tool to create your usual face. The same brush strokes practised every day leave products falling into the same creases: a different-sized brush will create a fresher look.

335 BRUSH-UP

Invest in good-quality make-up brushes, as these will make application easier, faster and more polished-looking. Brushes should always have bristles that feel soft against the skin. It's important to wash them at least every three months with a mild liquid soap.

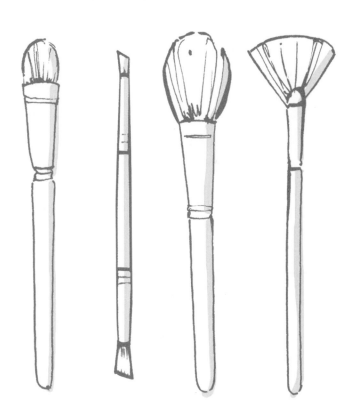

336 BARE-FACED CHIC

Unless you intend to spend the day tucked up in bed reading magazines, you should learn a basic skincare and make-up routine that suits you. As we age, our skin needs help to face the world. Presenting ourselves naked in the belief that bare-faced chic will help us look younger is a fallacy – it actually makes us look older.

337 DON'T BE A DISCO BABE

Better-quality products that contain finer ingredients are a wiser choice as we age. Products that are dazzlingly brash and bright, overloaded with glittery gels and coarser textures tend to look better on the young, and will almost certainly cause some irritation to delicate skin.

338 A SUMMER FACE

Summer make-up should be kept subtle. All you need are touches of colour to create a glow, and you should think in terms of eyes or lips, tempered with neutral blush and clear skin for fresh-faced summer beauty.

339 RUB-A-DUB-DAB

Always take make-up off at the end of a long evening because it will have combined with all sorts of irritants and pollutants, including airborne smoke particles, to form a suffocating layer over the skin. Gently dab with a cotton wool and never rub or pull at the skin.

340 HIGHLIGHT THE GOOD BITS

Draw attention to the bits of yourself you like the most. For example, if you have a round face, don't try to sculpt perfect cheekbones with make-up and too much blush. Instead, focus the attention on making your eyes the most dominant feature of your face.

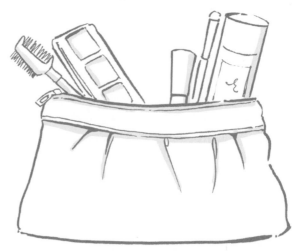

face base

341 NO SOLID FOUNDATIONS

Over-applying foundation in the belief that it will smooth away wrinkles is one of the most ageing make-up disasters. Use a light-textured foundation that will appear luminous on the skin and apply sparingly by patting it on rather than rubbing it in.

342 DON'T FORGET YOUR CLEAVAGE

When wearing a low-cut dress, remember to blend a light covering of foundation down from your neck and onto your chest, to give skin an even colour and smooth appearance. Always dust with a light covering of translucent powder to avoid getting foundation on your clothes.

343 BEAUTY IS SKIN DEEP

Good skin is always the basis for good make-up, so let it show by keeping the base sparse and not overloading it with foundation. Mix your usual foundation with moisturizer if it feels too heavy and mask-like on the skin.

344 FOUNDATION FAUX PAS

Wearing the wrong shade of foundation is instantly ageing – what you need is a perfect match to your skin. Test your base colour on your neck, near your hairline and next to your ear, then study the colour with a magnifying mirror in daylight. The foundation should disappear into your skin.

345 PRACTICE MAKES PERFECT

Use your fingertips, a damp sponge or a small brush to apply foundation. You will have to experiment to find out what looks the most natural. Whatever you use, never drag or pull foundation across your face – gently pat it into your skin.

346 A PERFECT MATCH

Ask for help at the beauty counter to find the perfect foundation colour for your skin, which will change throughout the year according to environmental factors, ageing and your own routine. Some of the better ranges will mix a colour specifically to match your skin tone.

347 BLUSHING BEAUTY

If you look pale and pasty, add a bit of warmth to your face with blusher. Choose a 'warm' or 'cool' tone depending on the colour of your skin. Apply blusher to the 'apples' of your cheeks – the most rounded part that rises up when you smile – and use sweeping, circular movements to blend the colour away to nothing.

348 BARELY THERE

Most people use far more foundation than they need: simply dot it onto the cheeks, forehead and nose and blend thoroughly. Don't be afraid to leave some areas bare.

349 CONSIDER YOUR SKIN TEXTURE

If you have large pores, apply your foundation with your fingertips. Applying it with a sponge tends to deposit too much, clogging the pores and making them more noticeable.

350 KEEPING IT LIGHT

Summer beauty requires a lighter touch. To keep your skin tone looking fresh and even, throw away your foundation and just use a tinted moisturizer with at least SPF 15 to cover the occasional blemish and also give you protection from the sun.

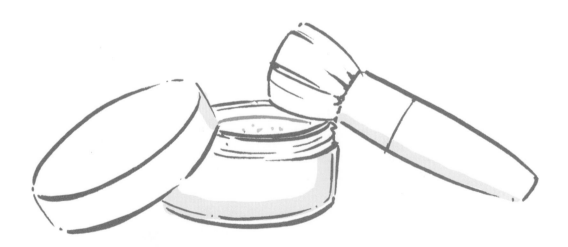

concealing & covering

351 BANISH BAGS

Lack of sleep is the primary cause of dark circles under the eyes. A quick-fix remedy is to apply a light-reflecting foundation in sequin-sized blobs under the eye. Using the index finger, blend gently into this very delicate skin.

352 PEP UP TIRED EYES

For very dark circles or hollow eyes, use a strong concealer and blend it in a little at a time with a concealer brush. Work by 'tapping' the concealer into the area rather than rubbing it into the skin.

353 REDUCE PUFFINESS

If you are plagued with puffy under-eye bags in the morning, use a botanical-based concealer formulated to cover dark circles and reduce puffiness at the same time. The formula should cool, firm and lighten the area all at once.

354 LITTLE IS BEST

Don't use foundation in an attempt to cover up deep creases and wrinkles; instead, use a highlighter sparingly to reflect the light and give your face a youthful glow.

355 KEEP A CORRECTOR PALETTE

When you wake up with dark circles under the eyes and a spotty blemished skin, reach for a corrector palette. A combination of yellow and green concealer targeted exactly on the glitch and blended in with a gentle finger massage will conceal a thousand and one problems.

356 DISGUISE ROSY RED CHEEKS

If you suffer from rosacea – excessive redness on the cheeks, nose, chin or forehead – use a green-toned concealer that will disguise the high colour. The concealer also has an ingredient that will improve circulation. If the condition worsens, you should consult your doctor or a dermatologist.

357 ZAP THOSE ZITS

Blemishes and spots may appear in the run-up to the menopause because of declining levels of the hormone oestrogen. Disguise them with a concealer containing salicylic acid to help reduce redness and blotches.

358 FOUNDATION FIRST

Apply your concealer after your foundation (if you are using any), as foundation may be all you need to conceal some blemishes. Blend it in with a brush or your finger.

359 DON'T GO LIGHTER

For concealing, don't go a shade lighter than your skin tone. This will only serve to emphasize the area. Using the same shade of your skin tone but with ingredients that are light-diffusing is a better choice.

360 HIDE THE TROUGHS AND WRINKLES

All make-up needs to be applied with a light touch: too much of any cream, liquid or powder will find its way into the tiny creases and wrinkles you are trying to disguise. Begin with just a tiny amount and add more as you need it.

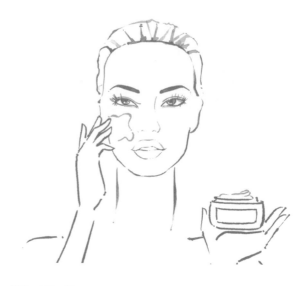

361 CONCEAL AND NOURISH

As we age, the skin becomes thinner under the eye area, and dark circles are more evident because the veins and blood vessels are closer to the surface here. This, combined with a genetic predisposition, is what causes dark circles to appear more prominent. As well as using a concealer, minimize the problem by moisturizing the area with an eye cream containing nourishing antioxidants that help protect the skin, such as green tea and grapeseed extracts, and vitamins C, E and K.

362 COVER UP AGE SPOTS

To keep skin an even tone, you need to cover up birthmarks, sun damage and age spots with a combination of foundation and concealer, using one or two shades blended together.

363 LOVE YOUR FACE

Learn to love your imperfections, as they are the defining things that make you special. Do not try to shade a nose with any type of concealer or shadow; it will make it look smudged with dirt.

364 TIP ABOUT CAPILLARIES

To cover up broken capillaries or an uneven skin tone, you can either massage concealer into the skin or paint the area with a brush, then blend it in with your fingertips.

365 CONCEAL BUT DON'T CAKE

Hide blemishes and red veins on fair skin with light-diffusing concealers that have peachy or yellow undertones. These are also brilliant at hiding under-eye shadows.

366 DON'T BE A SCARFACE

Even the most beautiful skin is susceptible to scarring over time, and no one reaches 40 without having some marks on their skin. To cover small scars, use a special dermatological concealer.

367 DE-PUFF DELICATE EYES

To provide a good base for your eye make-up, start with a good-quality eye cream to depuff and moisturize the delicate skin around your eyes.

368 BRIGHT EYES

For tired eyes that need an instant wake-up call, dot small circles of liquid foundation under the eye, and up over the eyelid. Blend in very gently with a brush or your little finger to conceal any dark lines, then line the lower lid with a white pencil. The effect is instantly brighter eyes.

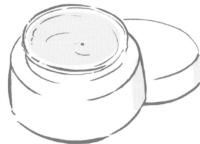

blushers & highlighters

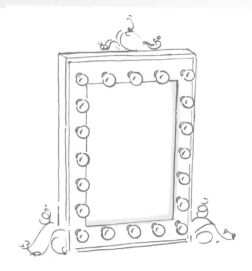

369 PALE AND BEAUTIFUL

If you have very pale colouring, stop wasting time with fake tans and bronzers – embrace your paleness and add a fresh-faced shade of blush to the apple of your cheeks where the colour naturally rises.

370 PROTECT WITH POWDER

A light, luminous powder can be useful in setting your make-up because it helps to lock in moisture to the skin, and protect it from environmental damage.

371 BRIGHTEN WITH HIGHLIGHTER

Add a little highlighter to brighten up pancake-flat skin, but always look for one with a very fine shimmer rather than garish sparkles, which can only ever look good on the very young. Blend over cheekbones and under eyebrows for a look that is glowing but not greasy. You can also mix it in with your usual foundation as a skin brightener.

372 IN THE SPOTLIGHT

If you want to know where to apply highlighter, stand in front of a mirror in bright light to test the best areas. As you are trying to achieve a natural-looking glow, you should only emphasize those areas that are directly hit by daylight, for example the tops of the cheekbones.

373 PLAN STRATEGICALLY

Give your face a cunning boost by dotting small dabs of highlighter in strategic spots – in the inner corners of the eyes, on the lips or on the tip of the nose – for extra shine and definition.

374 RADIANCE BOOSTING

Products sold as 'radiance boosters' or 'illuminators' usually have several roles. They can be used as highlighters to emphasize bone structure, as masks to revive lacklustre skin and eliminate fine lines, and under foundation to give a smooth surface, tighten the skin and provide glow.

375 SUN-KISSED

If you don't have time to apply fake tan, a cream bronzer will give the effect of sun-kissed skin. Use on the cheekbones, temples, down the bridge of the nose, and the centre of the neck for a glowing youthful complexion. Apply with a light touch for a natural look.

376 THE BEST BLUSHER BRUSH

Always choose a big blusher brush with a flat head and lots of densely packed bristles. Make sure, too, that it is made from 100% natural hair. This type of brush will be kind to your face and not scratch delicate skin, but more importantly it will apply blush and bronzer evenly without creating any ugly stripes.

377 AN INSTANT GLOW

Skin loses its pigment and colour as we grow older, so a quick brush of rosy blusher is most important, particularly in winter when skin is even paler. It will add an instant glow and make you look youthful and vibrant.

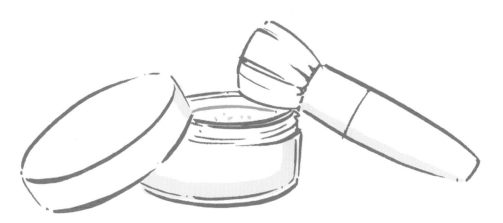

eye make-up

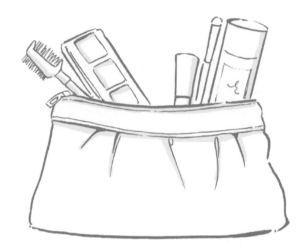

378 NATURALLY SOFT AND SHEER

Soft, neutral shades will help to open up eyes, while dark moody ones can make them look smaller and deep-set. Too much shimmer will settle into crease lines and reflect light, which will only draw attention to your crow's feet, so limit shimmer to the inner corner of the eyes.

379 SEMI-PERMANENT TIME-SAVER

A non-surgical treatment, semi-permanent make-up is implanted into the skin using an infusion of organic or mineral pigments. Adding stronger definition to the eyelids can save time and give an 'optical lift' to the eyes. Consult a recommended professional.

380 HEAVY METAL MAGIC

To brighten dark eyes, dot a tiny smudge of silver metallic shadow on the inside corner of the eye. This will give the effect of widening the eyes and making them sparkle.

381 SHADOW IS SOFTER

A smudgy eyeshadow line can be more flattering than a hard sweep of eyeliner. Blend the outer edges to create a softer look, which doesn't draw so much attention to the fine lines and creases around the eyes. Use a shadow powder and eyeliner brush rather than a pencil to push the shadow into the lash line.

382 CREAM SHADOW NOT POWDER

As the skin on our eyelids becomes dry and thin as we age, we need to choose a cream eyeshadow, not a powder one, because it will last longer on the eyelid.

383 FINAL TOUCH

When you've finished making up your eyes, put a tiny speck of iridescent colourless shadow onto the centre of your eyelid near the lashes. This will pick up light and make the eyes look wider and less hooded than they really are.

384 BROWN FOR BLONDES

If you are fair skinned and have natural or highlighted blonde hair, lay off the heavy black mascara, which will look unnatural and harsh. Blondes should always choose dark brown mascara, which suits their colouring much better.

385 NO-MASCARA LASHES

If you always end up with mascara running down your face by the end of the evening, think about having your lashes tinted and permed. Dark, curly lashes without layers of cloggy mascara will draw attention to your eyes in the best possible way.

386 GO ALL THE WAY

Whether you choose to use a smudgy soft eyeliner pencil or a liquid liner, always draw across the whole length of the upper eye. Just covering half of the top lid will make your eyes look smaller and more close-set.

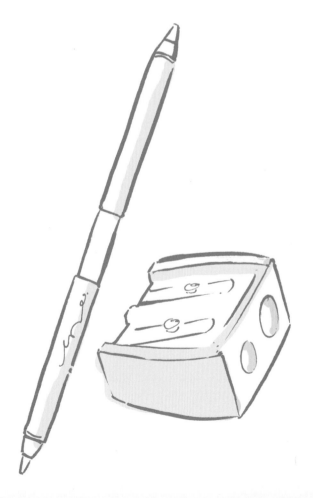

387 PERFECT EYELINER

Cheat a little and remove any wrinkle-created wobbles with a cotton bud (Q-tip) soaked in make-up remover. What you take off is as important as what you put on, and nobody will ever know that you cleaned up your mistakes to leave a perfect straight sweep of colour.

388 CREATE A CURL

Eyelash curlers really do help to open up your eyes, which can become less accentuated with age, and there seems to be little difference between the cheapest and more expensive ones. Curl your eyelashes before you apply mascara, as you are less likely to create clumps.

389 NO MORE CLOGGING

Sweep your mascara brush upwards in a generous curve to make lashes appear longer and thicker, but only brush the ends of the lashes and keep it away from the roots. Too much thick mascara around the base of the lashes will make eyes look small and narrow.

390 FLIRTY EYELASH EXTENSIONS

As hair starts to thin, some people notice their eyelashes fading, dropping out and almost disappearing. A recent process to add long, thick lashes to your own with a non-toxic bonding process allows synthetic lashes to be individually attached to each natural eyelash, for a fluttery, flirty effect.

391 FAKE IT

You can enhance the length of your natural lashes without ending up looking like a drag queen if you alternate the length of the fakes. Apply short and medium-sized fake lashes side by side for a special eye-opening party face.

392 DOUBLE-UP MASCARA AS LINER

For a quick but glamorous look when you only have a limited bag of make-up, use a loaded-up black mascara wand at the base of the lower lashes to create a flattering line along the lower eye. This quick trick will accentuate and open up the eye when you are caught without your usual eye pencil.

393 GO FOR LENGTH

If you tint your lashes to save time on making up with mascara, always use a clear gel mascara wand over top, which contains tiny fibres that lengthen your lashes, and make them look longer than they really are.

394 KEEP IT ALL UP TOP

If you often find your eyes look puffy underneath, keep make-up focused on the top of the lid. Avoid under-eye mascara if you're puffy because it tends to smudge, and shade only the upper eyes to make them look more open.

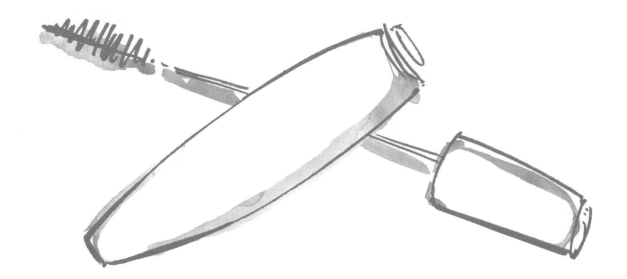

395 LESS SHADOW, BETTER RESULTS

Use eyeshadows sparingly, as eyelids become wrinkled and hooded as we age, and a heavy-handed application shadow will lie in creases along the wrinkles.

396 LASH-EXTENSION MASCARA

Ageing can leave you with shorter and lighter-coloured lashes. Find a mascara that has copper peptides listed in the ingredients – it is known to enrich hair follicles and make lashes longer.

brow shaping & colouring

397 TAMING CURLY BROWS

A tiny dab of petroleum jelly – or lip gloss, at a pinch – can help train curly hairs into a sleek, sophisticated line. Alternatively, use a little hairspray sprayed onto your eye brush to smooth them into place.

398 TAKE A BREAK

If overplucking or age has left your brows sparse, first try to resist tweezing them at all for a few months so you can see what you've really got to work with. Sometimes the habit of tweezing is so ingrained that you do it daily without realizing how much you're taking away. You may rediscover the natural beauty of your youthful brows.

399 FILLING IN OVERPLUCKED BROWS

Bald patches can be filled in by brushing the brows upwards and then filling in the sparse area with shadow powder that's a shade lighter than your natural brow colour. Finish by going over the area with a pencil that matches your brow colour, using short, hairlike strokes.

400 QUICK BROW LIFTS

Sweep a coloured brow gel over your brows as a last-minute beauty fix. It will tint the brows, as well as pulling straggly hairs into place. Tidy brows 'open up' small eyes.

401 THE PERFECT PLUCK FACELIFT

With age, the upper eyelids tend to sag
down, which is why a perfectly shaped
brow can act as an instant facelift. Decide
where you want to pluck by shading in
the area with a sweep of white eye pencil,
freeze the skin with an ice cube, and pluck
as close to the root of the hair as possible
only within this shaded area.

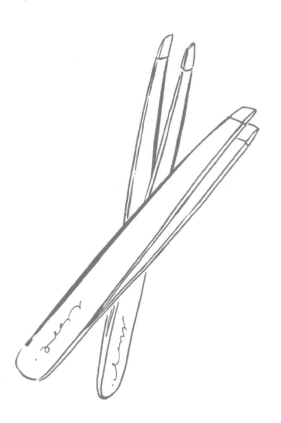

402 HELP FOR THIN BROWS

Hair thins on the brows as it does on the
head, so if you need to create the illusion
of fuller brows, use two colours of brow
colour or eyeshadow (never a pencil) –
a lighter one for the fullest part and a
darker one for the 'tails'. The shadow will
create a full, soft look that isn't possible
with a pencil.

403 DON'T LET YOUR BROWS AGE YOU

Brows that are too close together can
make you look old and frumpy. Never
artificially draw in your brow or try to copy
a celebrity's brows – the only brow shape
that will look good for you is your own
natural one.

404 GET IN PERFECT SHAPE

To work out how far your brows should
extend, hold a pencil vertically alongside
your nose to mark the inner edge of the
brow. For the outer corner, hold the pencil
diagonally from your nostril to the outside
edge of the eye. Pluck any stray hairs
beyond the pencil to open up your eyes.

405 COMBAT GREY BROWS

If your eyebrows are losing their colour, never attempt to darken them yourself with an over-the-counter dye, as it is all too easy to go too dark. Allow a professional to undertake the challenge, and between visits shade your brows in with a matching brow colour in a 'wand' applicator like mascara. As it simply washes off, there's no danger of a long-lasting mistake.

406 ENOUGH TO SHAPE

Eyebrows that are very thin can look quite ageing; stimulate growth in overplucked eyebrows by daily brushing very gently with an old, soft toothbrush.

407 SHAPELY EYEBROWS

It's best to combine different techniques to get the best shape possible. Waxing creates the overall shape and a defined outline, but small stray hairs should be plucked and trimmed to ensure a perfectly groomed eyebrow, which will define the shape of the face and open up tired eyes.

408 COLOURING IN

To make brows stronger in colour, use a combination of two different shades of eyebrow pencil, which will give a more natural look. Create a stippled effect with lots of tiny dots, rather than scribbling long lines over your brows.

409 FABULOUS THREADED BROWS

A traditional Indian beauty art, threading is a professional treatment that removes straggly brow hairs. The practitioner uses a length of thread to wrap around individual hairs and extract them from the root. The technique enables all the fine hairs to be removed too, which creates a cleaner-looking line. Threading is also used to remove unwanted hair on the upper lip and chin areas.

410 OVERNIGHT FIX

Brush eyebrows into shape every night using petroleum jelly. It encourages hairs to grow and leaves them thicker and glossier, making it easier to reshape into a perfect arch.

411 REJECT A PERMANENT BROW

Don't be tempted to have brows tattooed on permanently in order to save time and create a perfect line; the effect is hard and artificial.

lip cosmetics

412 INCREASE LIP VOLUME

Maximize your lip potential with volume-boosting lip gloss, which will increase the size of your lips and also help to reduce fine lines and wrinkles that form above the top lip. Lip-plumping gloss contains ingredients that react with the skin, resulting in fuller, plumper lips without the need for surgery.

413 PREVENT DRY LIPS

Always carry a lip balm in your handbag and remember to use it several times a day in cold harsh weather. Look for one containing shea butter or aloe vera to keep lips plump and hydrated.

414 DEFINE A FULLER LIP

As collagen production decreases, lips can lose their fullness. Small, thin lips can benefit from using a lip pencil that is the same colour as your lipstick. Define the full extent of your lips, and then blend the lip pencil with lipstick.

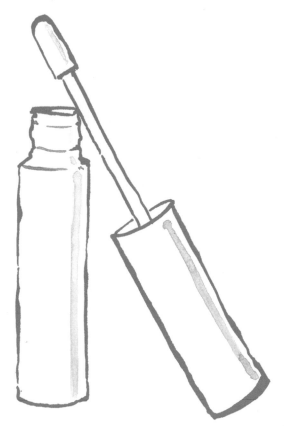

415 LEAVE OUT THE LIP LINER

If your lip colour has a tendency to
bleed upwards and outwards, apply a
moisturizing lipstick with your fingers in
small controlled daubs with your finger,
rather than 'dragging' the lipstick along
the mouth, which can look sculptured
and old-fashioned.

416 LIGHT TRICK LIPS

To give the illusion of a fuller upper lip,
dab a tiny touch of pale iridescent sheen
in the centre of the lips. This will highlight
your cupid's bow, making it appear bigger
than it is.

417 DARK LIP DISASTER

Unless you have a perfect pair of lips and
the expertise of a professional make-up
artist, very dark lips are best avoided. They
are ageing and unflattering on most faces,
as the contrast between lip colour and
skin is too dramatic, and the colour often
comes off on your teeth.

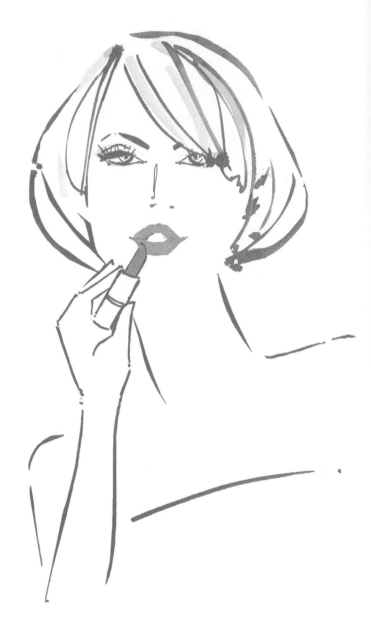

418 A LICK OF LIPSTICK

Resolve to find a flattering lipstick to keep with you at all times. Look for one that matches your natural lip colour but with a touch more zing. When you need to leave the house in a hurry, one swipe of this lipstick will give you instant polish.

419 SHEER LIGHTNESS

If you have a small mouth and thin lips, steer clear of dark, matt colours, which will make your mouth look meaner, and visually accentuate the flesh-coloured wrinkles that form around the lips. Instead, go for sheer, light colours of a similar shade to your natural lip colour.

420 FIX THOSE LIPS

Ruby red lips are too bold on an older face and tend to look cheap. If you do want to use a deep shade, make sure it doesn't 'bleed' into your wrinkle lines by using a transparent lip liner that will seal the colour.

421 CHOOSE A SUBTLE STAINER

As you get older, you lose the colour from your lips, so even if you prefer to wear nothing more than lip gloss or balm, you should prime lips with a subtle stain first to enhance your natural colour.

422 INSTANT COLOUR

Carry a neutral shade of lip gloss in your pocket. It is easy to apply in a hurry without a mirror using your fingertips, and will add instant colour and shine to dry lips.

423 MAKE TEETH WHITER

Choose your lipstick colour carefully; shades of purple or blue-based pinks can make teeth look whiter, while orangey browns will make them look yellowish.

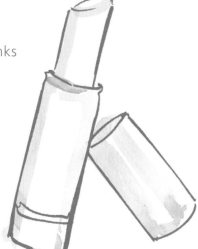

424 CHOOSING A LIPSTICK

Don't wear make-up when you go shopping for a new lipstick because then you can look at the true colour of your skin and lips and find a colour that suits your unmade-up skin tones.

425 PERFECT PARTY LIPS

When you're at a party and don't have time to keep re-touching your lipstick, use one that has a waxy base, which will stay put all evening and will not bleed into the fine lines around your mouth.

426 LONG-LASTING LIPS

The new formula long-lasting lipsticks that really stain lips are best avoided. They are hard to apply perfectly, will emphasize the shape and size of your lips and show every lip line that has formed around the mouth. Best to stick to neutral gloss and nude tints, which will make the most of what you have.

nails

427 QUICK-FIX SPLITS

Never leave the house with a tiny split or tear in your nails, as it is bound to develop into a ripped or broken nail with time. Use an over-the-counter nail-mender kit and apply a tiny strip of fibrous paper over the split before painting nail-mending liquid onto it and covering with polish.

428 NAILS HATE HARDENER

Prolonged use of nail hardener that contains formaldehyde will have a drying effect on nails and make them break more easily. To promote healthy growth, rub in equal portions of jojoba and vitamin E oil to cuticles and nails once a day.

429 ALWAYS ON SHOW

Well-groomed nails will always get noticed. Clear or pale pink varnish will give you a chic, finished look that is much better than long red talons, which are ageing and brash.

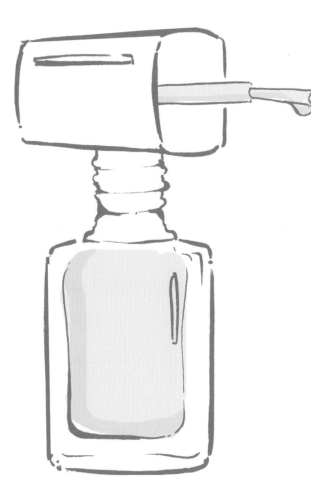

430 GORGEOUSLY GROOMED NAILS

The strongest types of artificial nail are acrylics and gels. The manicurist has to roughen up your own nail surface before painting over thin layers of liquid acrylic, which is extended up above your natural nail to the desired length. Easy to paint and strong enough to last for around three weeks, they make ugly hands look beautiful.

431 FEED NAILS FOR GROWTH

As you age, your nails grow at about half the rate they did when you were younger. Feed them by massaging a vitamin-rich oil into the base of the nails every night to encourage growth from the nail bed.

432 A BUFF TOO FAR

Nude nails that are clean, shiny and buffed are preferable to a single coat of chipped polish, but only buff nails once a week. Over-buffing weakens the nails by taking away the top layer, making them more porous.

433 LONGER-LOOKING NAILS

If you want to avoid having smudged and bleeding varnish, leave a margin around your nails when you are painting them. In addition, this will make your nails look longer and more elegant.

434 KEEP NAILS HYDRATED

The health of the nails and hair is very closely related to the overall health of the body. Keep the cuticle hydrated with specially formulated cuticle oil or a greasy lip balm, which can double up as an instant moisturizer.

435 FAKE IT

Don't let ugly broken toenails ruin your summer look when they will be constantly exposed in strappy sandals. Fake plastic nails that are glued onto your own nails at home and then shaped to the right size are perfect for toes that are unlikely to be inspected at close range.

436 SILK-WRAPPED NAILS

Try enhancing the length of your nails with silk fibreglass wraps that are glued onto the top of your own nail and then built up with layers of glue. When the nails are dry, they are buffed and polished for a natural effect, avoiding that fake plastic look.

437 BACK TO BASICS

To keep varnished nails healthy, you should always apply a base coat before applying polish. It helps the varnish bond to the nail and will prevent colour staining through onto the nail base.

super smiles

438 KEEP SMILING

Nothing is more attractive than a woman with a happy smile. It makes you look young, fun and carefree, so don't save your smile for special occasions – use it every day.

439 SHINY BRIGHT SMILES

As people grow older, their teeth become naturally darker, through smoking, staining and a build-up of tartar. Keep yours white with an over-the-counter kit containing a mild solution of hydrogen peroxide gel, which is rubbed into the teeth for about 30 minutes.

440 A PROFESSIONAL SMILE

A dentist can bleach your teeth externally using a custom-made rubber mouth guard and a bleaching gel. To achieve the colour you want, you need to wear the mouth guard with the gel for a few hours each day and continue the treatment for a few weeks at home.

441 HEALTHY GUMS

Poor oral hygiene will lead to gingivitis and eventually to teeth becoming loose and starting to separate. Daily plaque removal and thorough brushing with a fluoride toothpaste will help to maintain healthy teeth and gums.

442 LASER BLEACHING

The dentist uses a rubber seal to protect your gums, and then uses a special bright laser to shine on the bleaching gel. The laser speeds up the bleaching process and can make your teeth brighter.

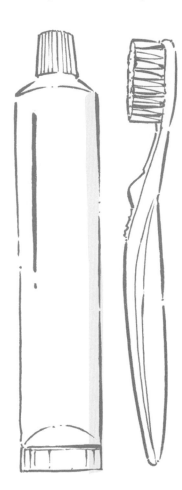

443 INSIDE-OUT BRIGHT

Internal bleaching places the bleaching product inside the tooth. The dentist will drill a hole in the tooth and put the product inside, sealing the hole with a temporary filling, and leaving the bleach inside the tooth. About a week later, the bleach is taken out, and the small hole filled.

444 BE WHITER AND BRIGHTER

Years of drinking coffee and tea and smoking cigarettes will leave your teeth yellow and stained. In addition to regular brushing, try mixing baking powder and lemon juice together, and gently massaging into teeth and gums for a natural way to whiten your teeth.

445 PERFECT PORCELAIN

If you feel let down by teeth that are crooked or chipped, consider having custom-made veneers for them. Formed from a thin shell of porcelain or composite material, they are cemented to the front side of the tooth and will leave you with a perfect set of shiny white gnashers.

446 STRAWBERRIES AND GLEAM

An inexpensive way to brighten teeth is to mash up a couple of strawberries and turn them into a paste to use as normal with a toothbrush. The malic acid in the fruit will help lighten your teeth – but always brush with a fluoride toothpaste immediately afterwards.

447 SPEED IT UP

For that Hollywood smile, you need straight, even teeth. A new method known as accelerated orthodontics can straighten your teeth and correct an overbite or underbite in three to eight months, rather than the traditional two or three years.

448 GET A LIFT

Oralift is a new antiageing dental brace that works by slightly widening the gap between the teeth which forces the muscles in your face to change shape slightly, boosting blood flow and rejuvenating its appearance by reducing wrinkles.

449 DENTAL FACELIFT

Specifically designed to counter the ageing process, the dental facelift restores both front and back teeth to their proper size using bonded porcelain. New teeth will support the jaw and restore proper facial dimensions, getting rid of deep mid-face creases and lines.

450 CAP IT WITH A CROWN

Cosmetic dentistry can work wonders for teeth that are poorly shaped, badly decayed or simply worn down with age. A dentist can fit perfect white crowns that have been made to fit over your whole tooth. When the whole mouth has been fitted, you will have a natural-looking set of perfect teeth.

451 SMILES BETTER WITH FLOSS

Flossing should be done once a day, ideally after the evening meal, to get rid of any small pieces of trapped food and to reduce plaque. Push the floss between the teeth and use a gentle sawing action. For bigger gaps between the teeth, use interdental brushes.

452 CHECK IN REGULARLY

Make regular appointments to see your dentist to keep a check on your overall oral health. Oral cancer, which is linked to smoking and drinking, is on the increase, and a dentist will be able to pick up on anything that is abnormal.

hair removal

453 SHADY LADY

Laser treatment is the best solution for removing dark hair growth on the upper lip. Choose a long-pulse laser (Alexandrite) in preference to the more common IPL (intense pulse light) for the most effective results.

454 WAX AWAY

Shadowy upper lips need to be treated regularly, and if you have dark colouring, it's best to get a hot-wax treatment at a salon. This will remove the small hairs instantly, but can be painful and will leave your skin temporarily irritated.

455 LOW-LEVEL ELECTROLYSIS

This treatment takes lots of time, is is painful but permanent. It must be performed by a qualified electrologist, who inserts a needle into the follicle and then sends an electric current to kill it. If performed badly, inflammation and scarring may occur.

456 CLOSE SHAVE

The fastest, most effective way to shave your legs is in the shower, with a clean, sharp women's razor. The hot steam opens the pores and ensures a close shave. It is recommended as the most efficient way by a host of supermodels.

457 DISSOLVING PROBLEMS

For facial hair, you will need to use a depilatory cream or gel specially formulated for this delicate area. Quick to work and inexpensive, these react with the protein structure of the hair, so that the hair dissolves and is removed from the skin's surface. However, they can irritate sensitive skin, so do a patch test first.

458 BARELY THERE

Those sensitive to wax may prefer 'sugaring' to remove unwanted body hair. The syrupy mixture is formed into a ball, flattened onto the skin, then quickly stripped away to pull hair from the shaft.

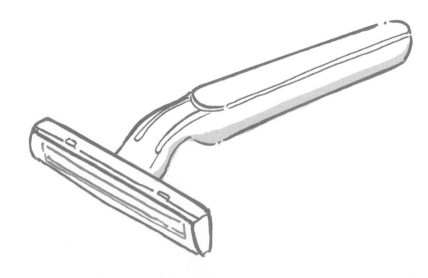

459 SMOOTH AND BARE

If you want to remove body hair on a long-term basis, try IPL (intense pulsed light) treatments. IPL devices rely on the absorption of light energy, which is targeted at the hair follicle, disabling it and preventing further growth. You will need several treatments, as hair has to be treated during its growing stage.

460 LASER BEAM REMOVAL

This treatment is best suited to light-skinned people with dark hair because the melanin pigment in the hair absorbs the laser light, making it more effective. The procedure causes the temperature within the hair shaft and follicle to rise, effectively killing it. Several treatments are needed to zap hair in its growing phase.

461 THE TROUBLE WITH STUBBLE

Hormonal changes in the body usually mean an increase in unwanted facial hair on the upper lip and sides of the face. Tweezers are brilliant for eyebrow plucking, but are much too severe to rip out these tiny facial hairs.

surgical body reshaping

462 GET PREPARED

If you decide to go for cosmetic surgery, it's very important to find a good surgeon and talk through any issues beforehand. Be realistic, too, about what surgery can achieve – it won't hold back the clock for ever but it will help you to age at your preferred rate. Your surgeon can advise you on what you need to do to prepare yourself, such as losing weight, stopping smoking, cutting out alcohol and taking extra doses of vitamin C.

463 RESIZE MY THIGHS

Losing weight may result in slack and saggy skin around your thighs that no amount of exercise will shift. Thigh-lift surgery is used to remove excess skin and fat from both the inside and the outside of the upper thigh, but the surgery will leave a noticeable scar around the groin.

464 TARGETING PROBLEM AREAS

Liposuction targets certain areas of the body where fatty deposits that are hard to shift have built up, like middle-aged tummies, hips and bottoms. New techniques are vastly improved, and 2–5 kg (5–10 lb) of fat and fluids can be removed at one time. For perfect results, skin needs to show some elasticity.

465 LOSE BOOB BULK

Breast reduction is a relatively simple operation for women who have large, heavy breasts that cause back and neck pain. Big boobs that are out of proportion to your size can make dressing difficult, and make you more self-conscious. An operation will leave you standing tall with less upper body bulk, and more confidence.

466 NO MIRACLE CURE

Liposuction can remove fat from beneath the skin and remove fatty deposits, and if you regain weight afterwards, it will mostly be in areas not suctioned. However, it cannot cure cellulite, tighten loose skin or take out fat from underneath muscles.

467 SLIM AND SEXY CALVES

New types of liposuction have refined the size of the suction tubes used to suck out fat, and this is revolutionizing the results that can be achieved on delicate areas like calves and ankles. Lower leg shape is often determined by muscle tone and underlying skeleton, so the results are often quite subtle.

468 PERK UP SAGGY BOOBS

Excess weight and the passage of time can cause breasts to droop and lose their shape. Breast uplift surgery can be done without altering the size of your bosom, as the surgeon simply makes a small incision around the breast to reposition the nipple higher and remove excess skin from below.

469 TINY TUCKS REDUCE BINGO WINGS

A hidden-scar arm lift (brachioplasty) removes excess skin and fat from the upper arms. A tiny incision is made in the armpit, and fat is removed from the upper arm while excess skin is pulled upwards towards the underarm, leaving arms firm and toned.

470 BOTTOMS AND THIGHS

After losing a lot of weight, you may find that you have loose, sagging skin around your buttocks and thighs, which no amount of exercise and healthy living will remedy. An operation can be done to raise and tighten the skin in these areas. If both thighs and buttocks are operated on, the procedure is known as a lower body lift. Cuts will be made in as unobtrusive a place as possible, and you will need to wear a compression garment after the operation to reduce swelling and to help to shrink and tighten the skin.

471 TUCK AWAY THAT TUMMY

A tummy tuck is not intended for weight control, but can be used for women who have excess skin and fat in their abdominal area, usually after substantial weight loss. An abdominoplasty requires the surgeon to make an incision across the bikini area, and then remove fat and skin; it will tighten the tummy muscles and leave the abdomen firmer and flatter.

472 SUPERSIZE ME

The type of breast implant – silicone or saline – plus the size and shape of your new bosom should all be carefully considered with your surgeon. The incision can be made under the arm, where it is hidden, around the nipple or under the breast. Full recovery time is about six weeks, and most implants have a lifetime guarantee.

473 LESS EXTREME THAN LIPOSUCTION

A new fat-busting treatment that is safer and less invasive than liposuction can suck fat from double chins as well as tighten up wobbly knees and bingo wings. Known as SmartLipo, the procedure uses a fine laser probe, which is inserted into the skin in the problem area to increase the temperature of the fat cells. This causes them to break down into liquid, which the body is then able to expel.

surgical facelifts

474 EARLY 40S FACELIFT

The most common procedures for people in this age group who want tightening in the face are performed with a shorter scar. The scar in front of the ear is a normal procedure, but behind the ear the scar is small and does not extend up into the scalp.

475 KNOW YOUR ZONES

In cosmetic surgery, the face is divided into three important horizontal zones, each one considered differently. The first is from the brows to the hairline where deep forehead furrows and brow lifts are done; the second is the eyelid to cheek area where crow's-feet and under-eye bags manifest; and the third is the lower face and neck area. Most facelifts target zones 1 and 2, as only subtle differences can be made to zone 3.

476 FACE UP TO A FACELIFT

There are several types of facelift that can be done to rejuvenate an ageing face, and the scars are designed to be well hidden. Skin at the temples, cheeks and neck is tightened upwards and backwards, and the layer of muscle tissue that lies underneath the skin (SMAS layer) is also treated in a similar way.

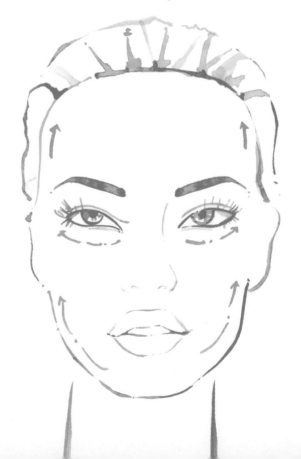

477 THE CUTANEOUS CUT

One of the first types of facelift that has been performed for many years, this relies on lifting the upper layer of skin only. Facial improvement occurs by lifting skin backwards and upwards, but there is no improvement to deeper facial muscles.

478 A LONGER-LASTING LIFT

Surgeons need to lift a deeper layer of skin to provide a longer-lasting result. By removing the soft tissues to which the muscles are attached (SMAS) and tightening them, or by lifting up a portion of the SMAS itself, it is possible to treat saggy jowls and redefine the neck.

479 A QUICK LIFT

The 'MACS' lift (minimal access cranial suspension) is good for patients with mild skin sagging, but no heavy folds around the neck. Permanent sutures are used to lift the soft facial tissue and suspend them in a more youthful position. There is a relatively quick recovery time, and a short scar behind the ears.

480 THE FAT INJECTION FACELIFT

Known as the Volumetric facelift, volume can be added to restore a youthful appearance. Fat from your own body can be injected into the face to plump up gauntness, and cheek tissue can be repositioned to the site it occupied before gravity produced its downward drift.

481 A BRAND NEW NECKLINE

Most neck lifts are performed at the same time as a deep plane facelift, the aim being to eliminate vertical folds in the neck, tighten the skin and reduce excess fat. The incisions are usually the same as for a facelift, although a small cut under the chin, known as a platysmaplasty, may be required.

482 UPLIFT DROOPY EYELIDS

Puffy, tired-looking eyes are usually caused by a combination of loose skin and excess fat. Common problems of 'hooded' eyes and bags can all be solved with eyelid surgery (blepharoplasty), which involves operating on the eyelid itself or removing and adjusting excess skin and fat.

484 BETTER BROW LIFTS

Keyhole surgery is on the increase to rejuvenate the forehead and lift the eyebrows. Ageing causes the brows to droop and look tired, which in turn causes horizontal creases in the forehead. New techniques for brow lifts keep incisions short (12–15 mm) and well hidden within the scalp, resulting in a fresher, more open appearance in the upper third of the face.

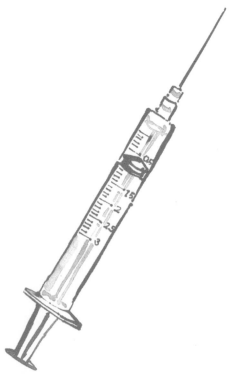

facial peels

484 A SUPERFICIAL LIGHT PEEL

Treatments that use alphahydroxy acids (AHAs) are light and will only remove the upper layer of skin. A series of peels is usually recommended, which will result in softer skin and the stimulation of cell and collagen production.

485 PEEL AWAY OLD SKIN

A chemical peel is simply an aggressive form of exfoliation that removes the top layer of the epidermis and all the flaws with it. The type of solution applied to the face, and the amount of time it stays on for, all determine how deep the peel is and how good the results are.

486 TARGET SPECIFIC PROBLEMS

A full facial dermabrasion treatment will incur a lot of swelling, and skin can look sore for up to 12 weeks, but the treatment is very useful for targeting trouble spots like specific scars or deep-set lines around the mouth.

487 DRYING-OUT SPOTS

A light glycolic acid peel will help to dry out patches of adult acne, dislodge blackheads and reduce shallow scarring, leaving your complexion brighter and softer. It makes skin more sensitive to UV radiation, so you will always need to use a non-irritating sun block.

488 OPERATION CROW'S-FEET

A medium peel using trichloroacetic acid (TCA) removes the epidermis and the upper layers of the dermis, penetrates more deeply than AHAs and requires a recovery time of about a week. Surface wrinkles, crow's-feet, minor scarring and small pre-cancerous moles are all suitable for this treatment.

489 SAND BLASTING

More aggressive than microdermabrasion or chemical peels, this procedure requires a specialist to 'sand' off the top layer of skin using a hand-held electrical device. When the new skin grows back, it will be smoother, less wrinkled and with all signs of sun spots or scarring reduced.

490 NONCHEMICAL PEELS

Microdermabrasion uses a high-powered combination of force plus suction to remove a very thin layer of skin, leaving only superficial wounds. Finely ground aluminium oxide or sodium crystals are blasted onto the skin, sloughing off the top layer, to reveal a fresh new layer underneath.

491 SKIN RESURFACING

Effective new techniques in skin resurfacing, designed to even out the surface and reduce pigmentation, can now be performed in your lunch hour at the beauty salon. The improvements can seem miraculous, but the treatments can be invasive and are not without risk, so you should not undergo any cosmetic procedure without good research.

492 RESURFACE THE EXTREMITIES

Light and medium peels can also be performed on the hands and the neck area to reduce visible scars and wrinkles, and help stimulate the production of new skin cells.

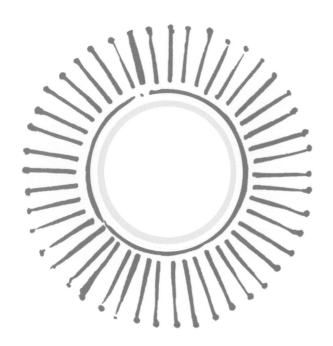

493 DEEPER EXFOLIATION NEEDS A HIGH DOSE

Phenol peels are more concentrated solutions of acid that are used to remove the epidermis and a large part of the dermis. As a treatment for deep facial wrinkles, areas of blotchy or sun-damaged skin and cancerous growths, phenol peels have proved to be very successful.

494 BETAHYDROXY ACID PEELS

A good alternative to an AHA peel, the betahydroxy peel has been found to be less irritating to the skin. As the salicylic acid involved is fat-soluble, the peel is able to penetrate oil-plugged pores and is therefore particularly suited to people who have active acne. Treatment may leave you with peeling skin for a few days, but it will remove blemishes and improve pigmentation.

495 PHENOL PEEL DOWNTIME

A full-face deep facial peel can take a couple of hours to perform and should always be done by a qualified dermatologist. The treatment can leave you in bandages for several days and looking red and sore for weeks, but severe wrinkling around the mouth and eyes will be dramatically improved and the benefits of the fresh new skin that emerges are long-lasting.

laser treatments

496 WHICH AREA TO TREAT?

For smoothing away wrinkles and resurfacing rough skin, lasers are best suited for three target areas of the face: the forehead and between the brows; the under-eye area extending to the crow's-feet; and around the mouth.

497 LUNCHTIME TREATMENTS

A 15-minute treatment with the N-Lite laser, which uses a specific yellow laser light to reduce wrinkles around the eyes and stimulate the growth of collagen, will leave your skin tingling, but you can put on make-up and go back to work straightaway.

498 NON-ABLATIVE LASER TREATMENT

Less intense than ablative treatments, this method stimulates new collagen production in the dermis, and causes skin contraction and tightening. The treatment essentially works by treating wrinkles from the inside out, rather than removing them from the outside.

499 ABLATIVE LASER TREATMENT

There are 3 types of ablative lasers used for resurfacing the skin: carbon dioxide (CO_2), erbium (Er: YAG); and the long-pulsed erbium (YAG). A qualified dermatologist will select the most appropriate treatment for you, but all focus laser energy on damaged surface layers and vaporize them, allowing collagen regeneration and new, smooth skin to grow.

500 MAGICAL LIGHT BEAMS

New laser treatments do not destroy outer tissue as they penetrate through to the layers beneath the epidermis to boost collagen production and improve skin texture, giving it a tighter and plumper appearance. The process is gradual and you will need multiple sessions to see results.

501 ZAP THOSE SPIDER VEINS

Treat tiny spider veins on your face with Intense Pulsed Light laser. This pain-free and non-invasive treatment sends light pulses into the cells causing the vein to collapse and then dissolve.

502 REJUVENATE WITH LASER

Thought to be one of the safest forms of cosmetic surgery, laser peeling offers more control in the depth of penetration and degree of precision for resurfacing problem areas of wrinkles around lips and eyes and specific scarring.

503 LASER LIGHT TO NEW SKIN

Fractional lasers such as Fraxel can resurface the skin in a non-aggressive way, making it softer, smoother and tighter. Using light sources that can stimulate collagen production and improve the appearance of fine lines, wrinkles, acne scars and age spots, there is no pain and the redness only lasts for 2–3 days.

cosmetic fillers & relaxers

504 PLUMP WITH COLLAGEN

Derived from bovine collagen (from cattle specifically reared for the purpose), this is one of the most commonly used fillers made to plump out laughter lines around the eyes and turn thin lips into voluptuous ones.

505 SALINE KISSES COMING SOON

Dermatologists are working on saline lip implants that will be inserted through tiny incisions along lip borders and then inflated with salt water, resulting in smooth but bigger lips.

506 LIP PLUMP

For a temporary lip implant and for people who cannot tolerate collagen, these hyaluronic acid gels are used with great success because they have the same chemical and molecular structure as an enzyme present in humans that helps keep skin moist and elastic.

507 FILL OUT WITH FAT TRANSFERS

Autologous fat transplantation plumps up skin using your own fat that has been liposuctioned from your thighs or abdomen. This can be used for deep lines, lip augmentation and acne scars.

508 NATURAL ALTERNATIVES FOR LAUGHTER LINES

Isologen and Autologen are two natural fillers made from your own skin cells that have been previously removed and allowed to incubate in test tubes until they produce collagen. There is no chance of an allergic reaction, and the injected treatment should last for up to two years.

509 SUPER GEL FILLS FACIAL LINES

A new man-made filler called Outline is being used to plump out the lines that form from nose to mouth. Made from tiny positively charged spheres, it attracts negatively charged molecules like a magnet, and instantly becomes part of your skin tissue. Results are instantaneous and can last for five years.

510 REMODEL WITH RADIO FREQUENCY

Skin tightening the jowly bits of the cheek that hang down below the jawline in ugly little bulges is now possible with a non-surgical procedure that involves radiofrequency remodelling. It contracts the skin that has stretched, giving it a lift and reducing the size of the jowls.

511 FILL THOSE WRINKLES

The technology to fill and reduce wrinkles is moving so quickly that there are now many different types of filler available. Synthetic and natural, injectable and non-injectable, permanent and temporary, all perform basically the same function, to plump up the skin and create a more youthful appearance.

512 SOFTFORM IMPLANTS

This synthetic hollow tube implant is used for smile lines around the mouth and frown lines, as well as to boost ageing lips. It is implanted beneath the skin and your own body's fibrous tissue grows through it, helping to keep the implant in place.

513 THE FACIAL FILLER DERMOLOGEN

Made from donor human cadaver skin, this treatment does not usually cause an allergic reaction, and is injected only into the area being treated, usually to augment lips and plump out laughter lines. It lasts longer than collagen, probably about six months before the implant is absorbed into the body.

514 BOYS MAKE COSMODERM

Scientists have been able to isolate and then replicate the collagen-producing cells found in newborn infant boys after circumcision. These can be injected into the skin to treat fine lines and wrinkles.

515 BANISH LINES WITH BOTOX

Botox injections containing the botulinum toxin have revolutionized antiageing treatments for the face. A tiny amount of the poison is injected into the skin, temporarily paralysing the muscles, which can no longer make the same expression. Lines are gradually smoothed and softened from lack of use. The areas it treats best are lines on the forehead and between the brows and crow's-feet.

516 NEW FILLERS TO LOOK FOR

Argiform, Dermalive and polyactic acid are all synthetic fillers that have been developed to inject safely into the face where wrinkles, folds and depression lines have formed over the years due to natural loss of moisture. They restore volume and leave the face looking smoother.

517 RESULTS WITH ARTECOLL

This filler combines bovine collagen with inert microscopic plastic 'beads' (less than the diameter of human hair), which become encapsulated by the body's own collagen, and therefore stay in place. It is used for lip enhancement, deeper wrinkles and soft facial scars.

518 A SAFETOX ALTERNATIVE

Safetox is an adhesive patch fixed to the forehead and worn with a plastic headband that releases electronic impulses onto the frown lines on your face. Safetox inhibits the muscles that create wrinkles; it activates and relaxes them, creating the appearance of a youthful and radiant face.

519 TYPE A TOXIN

The most potent and commonly used type of botulinum toxin is type A. The toxin attaches itself to the muscle where it was injected, so it cannot travel around the body and cause permanent damage. The effects should last for 3–6 months, by which time the body will naturally have destroyed the toxin.

520 BLOCK LINES WITH MYOBLOC

If your body has natural resistance to the botulinum toxin or you find it not strong enough to do the job, there is a larger dose called Myobloc, which is a botulinum toxin type B. The effects are a little more immediate and may last a little longer.

521 BETTER THAN BOTOX

A toxin called Xeomin, which works in the same way as Botox, is thought to have less chance of causing an allergic reaction because it doesn't contain the lab-produced foreign protein cells that are used as a carrier – so keep an eye open for this new 'Botox'.

522 THE NEW RADIANCE

Radiance (also known as Radiesse), a next-generation cosmetic filler, is an injectable paste made from a substance found in human bones and teeth. It can be used to fill laughter lines and folds, as well as being injected into lips to give a fuller pout.

523 RESTYLE WITH RESTYLANE

This dermal filler is made from hyaluronic acid, which, in turn, is derived from skin tissue. It has been used in more than 3 million treatments, restoring volume to the skin, which results in a smoother, more youthful appearance.

524 COMPUTERIZED FACELIFT

The science of Super TNS (Trophic Neuromuscular Stimulation) is designed to stimulate the foundation muscles of the face and body. The procedure will make skin look younger because of increased blood circulation, as well as enhancing tissue elasticity and lessening laughter and frown lines.

golden rules

525 DON'T DO MEENAGER (MIDDLE-AGED TEENAGER)

If teenage girls look good in 'it', chances are you won't. Nothing is more ageing than competing with young girls who have fresh faces and slimline bodies. Stay clear of their trends, skinny jeans, pierced belly button and exposed G-string, and choose clothes that suit your shape and colouring.

526 DRESS YOUR AGE

Fashion definitely becomes more about style and less about trends as you get older. Stay clear of anything that screams 'cute' and 'girly', such as puff sleeves, baby-doll smock tops or mini-dresses, or lots of ribbons or ruffles.

527 LESS IS MORE

Even if you consider yourself to be in good shape and well toned, you should never show off your breasts and vast expanses of bare leg. Make a choice of either one or the other, never both in the same outfit.

528 PURGE YOUR WARDROBE

Make a date to try on all your existing clothes in front of a full-length mirror. Assess yourself honestly and throw out anything that is unworn, old-fashioned, stained or simply too small. Everything that's left should make you feel fabulous when you put it on.

529 AVOID SLOBBING OUT

Fitted clothes are always preferable to shapeless oversized tents. Baggy clothes just hang from your widest point, do nothing to define your good points (everybody has one good asset) and make you look bigger. Elasticated waistbands don't work under any circumstances.

530 EMBRACE YOUR CURVINESS

Celebrate your womanly body by wearing clothes that show it off; bias-cut dresses, fitted waistlines and pencil skirts will suit you much better than trying to cover up under a loose kaftan. Wrap dresses are particularly good for the curvy figure.

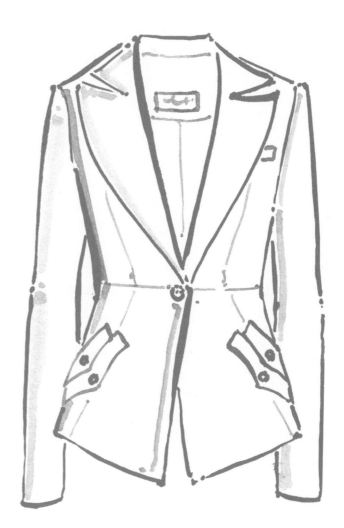

531 TOO MUCH CAN LOOK CHEAP

When finishing off your outfit, don't overdo it with accessories and end up looking ostentatious. If in doubt, leave it off. Learn to pare down your look so you know what suits you; learn what to add, and what to leave at home.

532 LEAVE HIS SHIRTS ALONE

At 16 it may be sexy to wear your boyfriend's shirt, but at 36 it will make you look like an old matron. Curvy girls with a bigger bust benefit from fitted shapes.

533 CREPEY CLEAVAGE

More than any other area, the skin between nipples and neck can provide a telltale giveaway to your age. Don't overdo the push-up bra or have a plunging décolletage, which will only highlight the problem of saggy parchment skin.

534 A HINT OF FLESH

Keeping arms and décolletage lightly covered with lace, chiffon or sheer organza keeps you from revealing too much flesh in the sexiest way possible.

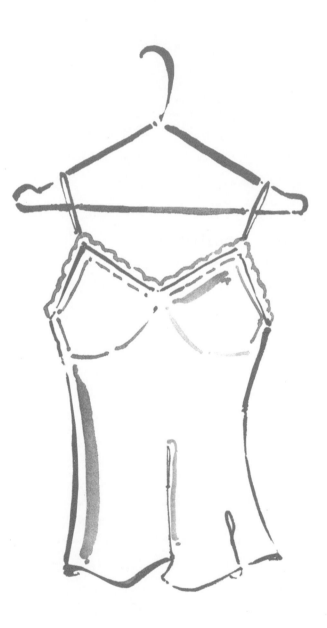

updating your wardrobe

535 SPEND TIME IN THE FITTING ROOM

Update your wardrobe every season with a few key pieces, and be prepared to try on a mountain of clothes to assess what you like. Following fashion from a suitable distance will keep you looking well groomed and modern.

536 MIX IT UP

High-street stores aimed at the very young can be great hunting grounds for the basics, but make sure you avoid the high-fashion items. Mix cheaper items in with your investment pieces to refresh your look.

537 DON'T GET STUCK

Matching every detail of an outfit makes you look dated, and choosing shoes, bag, earrings and necklace that all match is instantly ageing. Loosen up your style by wearing suit jackets, but not with the matching skirt or trousers, and choose from a colour palette where colours co-ordinate a shade or two away from each other.

538 THE PERFECT JACKET

An almost perennial classic that suits almost every shape and size if you tweak the proportion is the mannish-style jacket. A well-cut tailored suit jacket, single breasted without fussy detail, does a perfect job over trousers, dresses and skirts – if you get the length right.

539 AN ESSENTIAL PAIR OF JEANS

A good pair of jeans is a wardrobe staple for most women, who can easily take them from day to evening by changing shoes and shirt. You will need to spend time finding a good fit, and as a general rule, drainpipe skinny jeans flatter skinny minnies best and boot-cut jeans are much more flattering to all shapes and sizes.

540 NOT QUITE A CLASSIC

Fashion is in the business of changing shapes and styles, so look very carefully at old clothes that you bought as 'classic' investment pieces. Study the cut, lapel size, buttons, pockets and shape of an old favourite before you resurrect it. If the details aren't quite right, you will end up looking dated.

541 FIND A FEMALE ICON

Forget size 00 and teen fashion and find a stylish woman to copy. Choose a role model, like Helen Mirren or Bianca Jagger, who is roughly your shape and age, study the way they dress and steal their style.

542 CREATE A CAPSULE WARDROBE

Every season look for well-cut basic pieces to make a capsule wardrobe that will have some longevity and provide you with an outfit for every occasion. Versatility is the key, so find a dress that can be worn on its own or over trousers, and choose from a neutral colour palette of black, navy and stone.

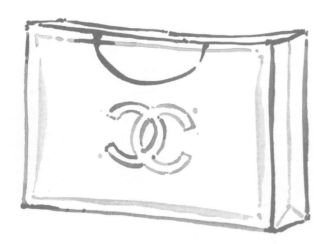

shopping strategies

543 PSYCH UP FOR SHOPPING

Prepare yourself before you hit the shops. Shop in the morning on a relatively empty stomach, and avoid 'bloat' days. Always wear seamless underwear, and take a pair of heels if the outfit requires them.

544 TAKE YOUR TIME

Never impulse-buy unless you find something you have been searching for and know it will be useful. Book yourself several hours off for shopping, and be prepared to try on lots of the same outfit. Always find a changing room with a three-way mirror so you can get a good overall view from every angle.

545 CHOOSE THE RIGHT SIZE

Make an honest assessment of your dress size, which is likely to change considerably throughout your adult life. Wearing clothes that strain across your shape is a definite style no-no, and will always make you look fatter, not thinner, than you are.

546 LOVE YOUR CLOTHES

Use wooden coat hangers for shirts, dresses and coats, and hang trousers by their hems from hangers with clamps. Misshapen clothes with lumpy wire marks will do nothing to boost your self-confidence and make you feel good.

547 THINK OUTFITS

It's much easier to shop for separates than for whole outfits, but always consider what the item you are buying will go with. There's no point in buying a fabulous organza shirt if you don't have a suitable skirt or trousers to complete the outfit. Try to think about matching things to your existing wardrobe to expand your choice, not individual pieces, which won't fit in.

548 SHOP ALONE

Shopping for clothes can be time-consuming, and having to accommodate a bored boyfriend or husband into the equation can be disastrous. Even a best friend can skew the agenda, so shop alone and trust your gut instinct when you try things on.

549 BUY BIGGER

A common mistake is to buy clothes too small, as psychologically squeezing yourself into clothes you wore at 24 makes you feel younger and thinner. It doesn't work. Choosing the right size of clothes will give you a better fit, accommodate curves where you have them and stop the fabric from straining.

550 GET A PROFESSIONAL STYLIST

A new career, divorce or just a change of circumstances can leave you floundering on the fashion front. If you have lost confidence about your looks, or really don't know what suits you any more, book an appointment with a personal stylist at a department store. The service is usually free.

551 TRY ON DIFFERENT SIZES

Make sure that all your clothes fit properly, and try on a larger and a smaller size to be sure. Choosing items that are too large will hide your actual figure and give the illusion that you are carrying extra weight.

552 THE OVERALL PICTURE

If you are serious about shopping, you should take armfuls of clothes into the changing room at any one time, and try pieces on that together make up an outfit. It's much easier to get an overall impression of a new wrap-around top if the bottom half looks right.

553 WHEN SIZE MATTERS

Every retailer will size their clothes for a slightly different fit, and there is no such thing as a standard dress size. Don't only try on one size; take the size above and below what you think you are, and see how they fit. Sizing can be inconsistent, so judge by how the garment feels and falls on your body, not by the label.

554 ASYMMETRIC SPLASH

Perfect symmetry, coiffed hair and designer dressing are boring. Our brains and eye movements are trained to skip over forms that are perfectly symmetrical, so if you want to make an entrance or grab someone's attention, dress and decorate yourself in an asymmetric style.

555 CHOOSE VINTAGE WISELY

Movie stars have the confidence to pull off vintage dressing, but for everyone else a secondhand piece from a charity shop can leave you looking like a frump. However, good vintage finds to look for, which can help you create a unique style, are accessories, quirky hats, silk scarves or an amazing handbag.

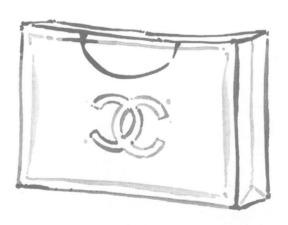

556 WISE BUYS

Never buy anything in a sale simply because it has been dramatically reduced in price, and never buy anything that will fit you once you have lost 2–3 kg (5 lb). Clothes have to fit properly, look good and make you feel great in order to be worth buying.

557 KNOW YOUR NAMES

Get to know the designers who make clothes that suit your figure and lifestyle. Betty Jackson, Nicole Farhi and Issey Miyake all produce understated collections with a sophisticated twist that perfectly fill the post-30-year-old wardrobe.

foundations

558 THE RIGHT FIT

Research has shown that 80% of women wear the wrong bra size. A good-fitting bra is supportive and uplifting as well as sexy, so get professional help in measuring and choosing the correct size.

559 UPLIFT YOUR LOOK

One of the narrowest areas on a woman's body is across the ribs, just beneath the bustline, yet sagging breasts can conceal this area and make your figure look dumpier and more middle-aged than it really is. Choosing a well-fitted bra with good uplift will help make the line from rib to hip appear more elongated and shapely.

560 BOOST YOUR ASSETS

Look for underwear that is appropriate for the job – one bra will not suffice for all occasions. To make the most of what you have up top, you will need a seamless bra for T-shirts, a strapless bra for evening wear, a sports bra for working out, and so on. All of them need to fit properly and provide firm support.

561 CREATE AN HOURGLASS FIGURE

Old-fashioned, all-in-one corsets are now available in comfortable Lycra. Not only will they iron out tummy bulges, but they will also enhance curves by lifting the bosom and creating a feminine waistline.

562 FIT YOUR BRA TO YOUR CLOTHES

When you are buying a bra, consider the clothes you will be wearing with it and bring them along if necessary. This is the only way you'll be sure that the bra fits the clothes. Keep an eye out for T-shirt bras, plunging bras, and labels that give an indication of the purpose the bra is made for.

563 PULL IN AND PUSH UP

Be prepared to try on lots of different styles to make the most of your assets. Every brand name measures slightly differently, so if you get measured for the brand you like, then you can buy others without trying them on. A well-fitting bra not only supports and lifts the breasts but also adds definition to the waist.

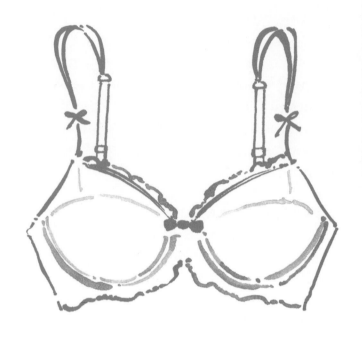

564 MORE UP TOP WITHOUT SURGERY

Silicone breast enhancers, commonly known as 'chicken fillets' because of similarities in colour, shape and texture to the real thing, are a great way to boost a flagging cleavage. Worn inside your bra, these fleshy gel sacks give the appearance of a fuller size and shape bust.

565 WHAT LIES BENEATH

If you need a good support bra to make the best of what you've got, shop around for something that is also eye-catching and pretty and will make you feel attractive every time you put it on. Frumpy grey nylon never made anyone's heartbeat miss a beat.

566 SAY NO TO VISIBLE UNDERWEAR

Under all circumstances it is best to avoid showing off your underwear during the day. If you are comfortably rounded, visible bra straps will push into your skin and leave unattractive bulges on either side, and the style of deliberately showing off a pretty bra strap or thong is best left to teenagers.

567 DROP A DRESS SIZE

Look slimmer and feel sexier with body-controlled underwear that can target specific problem areas. Seamless in construction, they come in all sorts of colours and shapes, from corsets to cycling-short underwear, and will enhance curves and banish ugly lumps.

568 LYCRA ALERT!

Don't be tempted to squeeze yourself into a bra that is too small, thinking that it will give you a greater cleavage, or choose smaller undies than you normally wear, believing that you will look even slimmer. Blobby rolls of flesh will be pushed out and be on show, defeating the point of the controlled silhouette.

569 TIGHTS THAT SLIM AND TONE

Look for very sheer tights that have a high quantity of elastane that will 'lift' your knees and legs. Designed to give some level of compression, these tights will improve your figure and 'slim' the look of the whole leg.

570 HELP FOR BIG BOTTOMS

Sexy undies come in all shapes and sizes, but if you have a full peachy bottom, don't overexpose it with a G-string. Instead, choose bigger, 1950s-style stretch shorts. Made in lacy Lycra and sheer tulle, they are ultra-flattering for bigger bottoms, and will smooth out bumps.

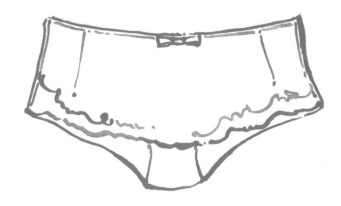

571 MAGIC KNICKERS

Look instantly slimmer with tummy-, bottom- and thigh-toning knickers. Made from a firmly holding stretch fabric that contains elastane, Lycra and polyamide, these comfy undies are designed to smooth out lumps and bumps and pull you into shape in all the right places.

572 NEVER UNDERESTIMATE UNDERWEAR

Great underwear is the foundation stone of looking good and feeling sexy. One size does not fit all, so get properly measured and fitted and choose the appropriate undergarment for each outfit.

573 WEAR YOUR BRA WELL

Many women fasten their bras at the front and then move them around to the back, but putting your bra on correctly can make a big difference to the way you look. First, hold the cups under your bust and bend forwards to let your breasts fall into the cups, and then fasten at the back before pulling the straps up. This cradles your breasts and places them exactly where they were designed to go, without pinching or squeezing anywhere.

trousers

574 THROW OUT THE CARGO TROUSERS

Slouchy combat trousers with huge saddlebag pockets add extra inches to your thighs and hips, so dump them in the charity box unless you have the physique of a supermodel.

575 CITY SHORTS

If you choose to wear smart city shorts as an alternative to a skirt in the summer, follow the rules. Apart from on the beach, shorts should always end on the knee and never above, and legs should be in good condition (tanned and hair-free). Always wear them with a small heel or wedge.

576 TURN-UPS ARE A TURN OFF

Trousers with a turn-up (cuff) hem and rolled-up jeans make the legs look shorter than they really are. Turn-ups attract the eye downwards to the detail, emphasizing any lack of inches in the leg department. Capris and wide gaucho trousers are also best avoided unless you have fabulous long legs.

577 HIDE AWAY FROM HIGH-WAISTERS

Look for jeans and trousers that are low-waisted, or sit between the hips and the waist. High-waisted trousers that clamp the middle tummy can highlight a lack of waist and accentuate any middle-aged spread. Even on the slim, they can push out abdominal flesh to create rolls of flab.

578 STAY AWAY FROM PATTERN

As a general rule, prints, patterns, checks and stripes will all emphasize bulging hips, bottoms and thighs. Plain-coloured trousers with a very fine pinstripe are a much safer bet. Never choose jeans that are embellished with diamanté beads, sequins, embroidery or fringing; these belong in Dolly Parton's Vegas wardrobe.

579 FLIMSY FABRICS SHOW IT ALL

If you are a classic pear shape with big hips and bottom, you need to find well-cut trousers made from a good-quality fabric that has some weight and body. Flimsy cottons and lightweight fabrics will show every bottom bulge and highlight problem areas, such as cellulite.

580 EASY LEG LENGTHENER

Add a little extra length to your legs by always wearing trousers that cover the top of your shoe and skim the floor.

581 PEAR-SHAPED BOTTOMS

If you have a pear-shaped bottom, you can still wear trousers as long as they are well cut, and not so tight that the fabric strains. Hipster trousers avoid the gaping waist problem, and will help to make your bottom look smaller.

582 TUMMY TRICKS

Many women end up with an extra roll of 'spread' around their tummy, but they can still look good in trousers, provided they choose flat-fronted ones with a side zip, which doesn't add any bulk at the front.

583 STRETCH AND SLIM

Keep a look out for good-quality denim that has a small amount of stretch in it, which will help to keep the jeans in good shape. Slightly thicker denim controls your contours and will make your legs look slimmer.

skirts & dresses

584 KEEP THE LENGTH LONGER

To disguise a general fullness around the tummy and hips, you need to keep skirt lengths to at least below the knee, or longer to mid-calf. Cutting off above the knee will visually keep you short and emphasize bulk, rather than drawing the eye down to elongate the body.

585 A SKIRT THAT WORKS FOR YOU

If you have good calves and ankles, show them off with a shapely pencil skirt rather than something flouncy. If you have crepey knees, choose a style that covers them. The effect is just as sexy.

586 DRESS TO IMPRESS

Look at your good points and dress to accentuate all of them. If you are curvy, choose a dress that's cut to fit the curves and not cover them, and if you have a fabulous cleavage, find a dress with a row of buttons that leads the eye towards it.

587 PLEATS ADD POUNDS

If you have a round physique and tend to carry weight around your tummy, choose a slim-fitted skirt. Fullness gathered into a waistband and knife-edge pleats that splay out will only emphasize your girth.

588 BIG BUST TACTICS

Wrap tops and dresses are great for defining and separating a big bust, provided you are wearing supportive (and the right-sized) underwear. A wrap dress can also emphasize a good waistline.

589 WRAP-AROUND WAIST

A big tummy benefits from a skirt that wraps around the tummy and has a tie-up side fastening. This allows the dress to be individually adjusted to make it smooth and flat without pulling or wrinkling.

590 DISGUISE THE SADDLEBAGS

If you want to minimize the appearance of bulky hips and a large bottom, choose a skirt that flares out with an uneven hemline. This draws attention to the hem and away from the saddlebags.

581 COVER UP BINGO WINGS

Short fitted cardigans and shrugs are perfect cover-ups to wear over any strapless or spaghetti-strapped dress to keep flabby upper arms in check. Look for those with three-quarter-length sleeves.

582 SHOW OFF AN ATTRACTIVE BACK

Instead of choosing to show a crepey cleavage, find a dress with a high slash neck that has a low sweep or V-neck at the back. Skin on the back has usually had far less exposure than that on the front and doesn't age nearly as much.

583 A-LINES FOR A BETTER BOTTOM

If your derrière is on the large size, stay clear of flouncy fashion statements like the puffball or tulip skirt, which both have too much volume. Buy an A-line skirt, which is the most flattering shape to cover up your figure flaw.

tops & knitwear

584 WALK TALL

If you suffer from a rounded back and slumped-over shoulders, invest in a small pair of shoulder pads to slip under your clothes. These will trick the eye into visually squaring off shoulders and will balance out wide hips.

585 SCOOP IT OUT

If your décolletage is lined or crepey, avoid wearing a deep scoop neckline that will expose a large expanse of skin. Also, bear in mind that the sweeping shape will draw attention to a low-slung heavy bosom.

586 RUCHING CAN FLATTER

Wear a ruched or gathered top with a zip or buttons up the front, which can form a V-neck while retaining the soft shaping. The soft gathers make a great disguise of unwanted lumps and bumps, and the V-shape will elongate the body.

597 STICK TO LONG SLEEVES

Even if you work out and have arms that are toned like Madonna's, skinny vest tops are best left for the gym. A scoop-necked top with bare arms will reveal too much flesh, and it's always more attractive to cover up with something sheer, which gives a suggestion of flesh but keeps it under wraps.

598 NECKLINES THAT FLATTER

Big-bottomed girls should look for slash-neck tops. A wide boatneck T-shirt will visually even out the width of your hips, and make you look more balanced.

599 SEXY SWEATERS

Sweater dressing for curvaceous bodies needs to be handled with care. Choose fine knits over thick chunky knits, which will add another layer of bulk, and choose a V-neck shape rather than a polo neck (which creates a no-neck look).

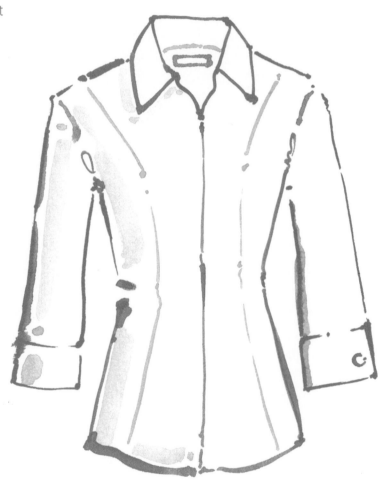

600 HEAVY UPPER ARMS

Choose a three-quarter-length sleeve top to camouflage flabby upper arms, and leave your elegant wrists and well-manicured hands on show.

601 A GREAT BARE BACK

If you have well-toned arms and good shoulders, wear a halterneck top (with a well-fitting halterneck bra underneath). A sexy back is just as alluring as a prominent cleavage.

602 GET A WIDE V-SHAPE

Big boobs benefit from a wide V-neck that cuts from the edge of the shoulders. This gives the effect of lifting and separating the breasts, but also draws attention upwards toward the neck and face, without covering up your assets.

jackets & coats

603 A HIP WAY TO DRESS

To minimize figure flaws, always draw attention away from the problem. If you have a big bottom and wide hips, stay clear of tiny jackets that cut off at the waist, and choose something longer, to mid-thigh, to cover the problem area. Always balance out your heaviest point.

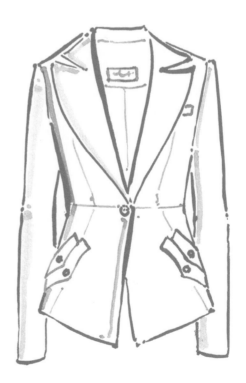

604 SINGLE-BREASTED IS BEST

As gravity takes its toll, and a layer of middle-aged spread appears around the core body, it's time to kiss goodbye to all double-breasted jackets. Always choose single-breasted coats, as two sets of buttons make the body appear wider.

605 BUTTONING-UP ADDS BULK

If you are broad-shouldered and busty up top, look for jackets and coats that have a V-neck and V-shaped revere; mandarin collars and buttons that extend up to the neckline will make you look bulky and square-shaped.

606 A COAT TO COVER UP

A fabulous coat can be thrown on over anything and instantly pull a look together. If you have the height to carry off a full-length coat, it can look wonderfully dramatic and will work equally well over jeans and flat boots as with high heels and a party dress. If you are petite, a long coat will only make you look shorter.

607 CREATING CURVES

If the ageing process has left you with a solid, boxy torso, you should create an optical illusion of feminine curves with a jacket that has a nipped-in waist and a flared cut or a peplum.

608 GREAT LENGTHS

The most versatile coat length is probably the three-quarter-length one that falls to just above the knee. It suits most figures, can be thrown on over any outfit and will cover a multitude of sins.

colour choices

608 CHOOSE COLOUR CAREFULLY

Our skin tone, hair and eye colour all fade as we get older due to loss of pigment and for that reason it's important to constantly reassess what colours suit us. Hold coloured fabric up towards your face in daylight to see which hues flatter you; avoid those that make your skin look sallow and drained.

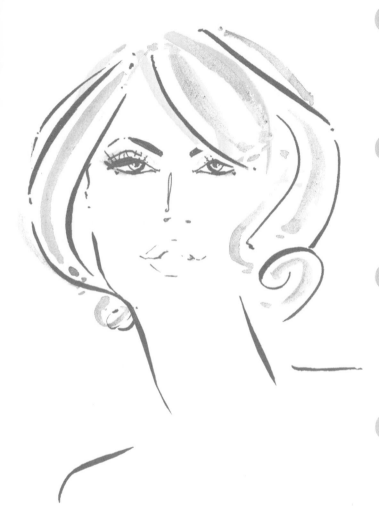

610 SHAPE A LEG

You can't go far wrong with black opaque tights, whatever the fashion. They slim the legs, making them look longer and leaner, and go with most outfits.

611 ACCENTUATE THE POSITVE

Always put colour and pattern on the parts of the body that you want to be noticed. Dark solid colours will camouflage figure flaws and draw the eye away from them.

612 THE LBD WARDROBE ESSENTIAL

Black may have a slimming effect but it also drains the colour from your face and can make you look old. If you want to wear a dark colour, navy blue or brown are both more flattering to older skin tones.

613 DRAINING AWAY COLOUR

Avoid dressing head to toe in black, as it is not only funereal and ageing, but it will also emphasize a sallow complexion. Black worn with acid brights is also a bad colour combo, and often ends up looking cheap and tarty.

614 TRICKS WITH TEXTURE AND COLOUR

If you want to play down a part of your body that you dislike, such as heavy boobs or thunderous thighs, it's always best to choose dark colours and matt fabrics. These avoid reflected light, which will make something look bigger than it really is.

615 BRIGHTEN UP YOUR OUTFIT

Forget the dictates of fashion and add some colour to your basic wardrobe staples. Choosing to wear a miserable selection of black, grey and beige every day can sometimes feed into emotions of sadness and depression. .

616 CREATE HEIGHT

Trick the eye into thinking you are taller and slimmer than you are by sticking with one colour choice for your bottom half. Brown trousers and brown shoes are visually seamless, whereas black trousers and beige boots crop the leg at the ankle and draw the eye downwards to the cut-off point.

617 DARK DENIM FLATTERS

No matter what body shape you are, choosing a great pair of jeans is possible provided you are prepared to take an armful of different styles and sizes into the changing room. Avoid pale bleached denim and opt instead for dark denim or black jeans.

618 RESIST THE ALLURE OF YELLOW

With age comes a slightly more 'washed-out' complexion, and any shade of yellow – from pale primrose to bright banana – will not look flattering on white skins. Black skins, however, look great with vibrant colours, even with age.

619 WHITE TOO BRIGHT

Super-dazzling white is too harsh a colour to wear for a complete outfit, and white jeans are a fashion no-no unless they are worn in the summer with a floaty kaftan over the top. Older women will find that a softer magnolia cream or ivory is much more flattering to skin tones, and will make an equally impressive statement.

620 NAVY IS CHIC

As an alternative to black, every shade of dark blue, from navy to deep azure, can look just as chic. Blue is a softer colour, so it is kind to mature skin that may have lost some of its lustre.

621 FISHNETS LOOK FANTASTIC

If you have a shapely pair of legs, fishnet tights can look fabulous, as long as you stick to black and choose the more flattering narrow weaves, not the pole-dancing types.

it's all about the fabric

622 SKIM BUT DON'T CLING

Fabrics that hug the body, such as cotton and silk jersey, are perfect for feminine curvy bodies, but they should always skim across the curves rather than cling.

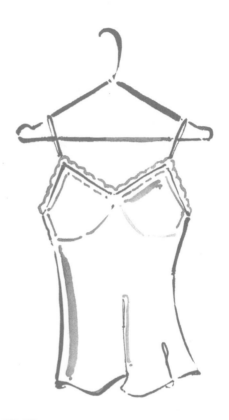

623 LAYERS CAN LOOK LUMPY

If your body has given way to gravity a little, be cautious with layering. A combination of different patterns and textures may make you appear shorter and fatter. Avoid outfits that cut across the body with lots of different horizontal layers or stripes.

624 LAYERS THAT SKIM

If your body shape is slim but less defined than it was, wear loose layers that skim your waist and cut off at the hips or mid-thigh. Belted trousers and tucked-in shirts will emphasize what you do not have.

625 LOOK FOR LINING

Where possible, choose skirts and trousers that are fully lined, as this helps create a much smoother line.

626 BEAT THE SWEATS

If you are prone to hot sweats, be sure to choose natural fabrics, such as cotton, rayon and silk. Stay away from synthetic fabrics that cannot 'breathe', like nylon and polyester.

627 LOOK FOR LINEN BLENDS

For summer, invest in a cool linen trouser suit, but instead of buying 100% linen, inspect the label to find a linen and silk mix. This blend will give you all the comfort and style of linen but will keep you looking polished for longer, as it produces fewer creases and wrinkles.

628 PATTERN DISGUISE

Learn which type of patterns will flatter your size, and which will emphasize it. A small-framed body will be drowned by huge OTT prints. Likewise, a larger lady should stay clear of tiny delicate prints, which will simply get lost on her frame.

629 CHOOSE CASHMERE

The ultimate comfortable and stylish fabric is cashmere, which is also warmer, softer and lighter than all other natural fibres. If you can afford it, choose cashmere above lambswool in winter because it has fantastic insulating properties.

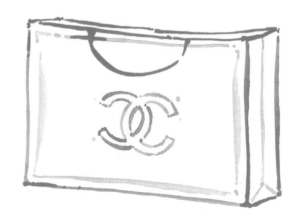

shoes

630 THE IDEAL HEEL

Find the most flattering heel shape to complement your leg shape. If you have slim and shapely ankles, a tapered slim heel will reflect this visually, whereas thick ankles benefit from a more sturdy, straight heel.

631 SECRET COMFORT CUSHIONS

If you know you have a long night of dancing ahead of you, slip a pair of silicone gel comfort cushions into your party shoes; the torture of wearing killer heels for hours on end will be dramatically reduced.

632 BOOTYLICIOUS!

If you like wearing knee-high boots over jeans or with knee-length skirts, choose a pair without fussy detailing in dark brown or black. A flattering pair of boots can slim ankles and visually lengthen the leg.

633 INVEST IN THE BEST

Good-quality shoes and boots speak volumes about you and the way you present yourself. It is far better to have one pair of truly chic shoes and one pair of fabulous boots than dozens of pairs of old styles that have seen better days. Make sure your shoes are always clean, and store them in boxes, so they are always in perfect condition to slip on.

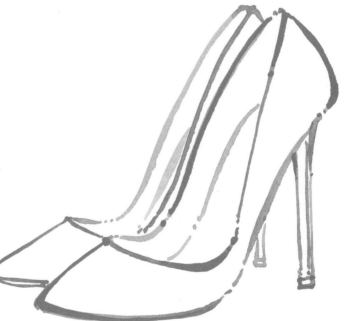

634 BEAT BORING BLACK

Get out of the habit of wearing the same black court shoes with every outfit. Old-fashioned shoes can date an outfit quickly, as the shape and size of the heel and the distinct shape of the toe change from season to season. Buy at least two new pairs of shoes every six months.

635 WHY WEDGES WORK

If you are petite, wear wedges instead of killer stilettos. They will give you a little more height but lots more stability. They are a less obvious choice than high heels and are more comfortable to wear for long periods of time or when you need to walk long distances.

636 WALK WITH CONFIDENCE

Heels that are too high to walk comfortably in will not give you enough confidence when you walk into a room. Small heels will improve the way you walk without the worry of ankle twists or falls.

637 SHOES FOR SHORTIES

If you are a little short in the leg, always choose shoes that have an open front to reveal as much foot as possible. Ribbons, laces and ankle straps visually shorten your leg length.

638 THE RIGHT SIZE OF HEEL

Shoes can help give the appearance of a taller, slimmer silhouette and a better posture. Flat shoes can be clumsy and make you more flat-footed, while high stilettos make you totter. A medium-sized heel will do wonders for the way you hold yourself.

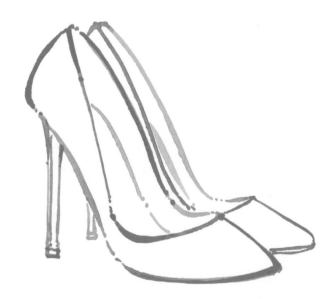

special occasion styles

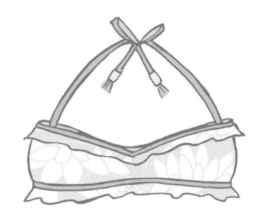

639 STOP SUMMER SWEATING

If you dread the thought of summer dressing because of telltale under-arm stains, invest in sweat pads, which stick easily into the armpit area of your clothes and stop dampness coming through.

640 LADYLIKE STYLE

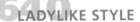

Many swimwear manufacturers are creating stylish collections of resortwear and cruisewear that appeal to the well-heeled woman. In many cases, these offer better support and coverage than those for a younger market, yet are still cutting-edge in the fashion stakes. Look at the catwalk collections for ideas from couture.

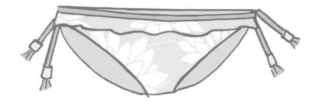

641 FLATTERING SWIMSUITS

If you want to draw attention away from big hips, choose a strapless swimsuit. The eye will be drawn to the strong horizontal line that covers the bosoms and upwards towards the shoulders and face.

642 SARONG STYLE

Take several styles of sarong, kaftan and cover-up on holiday with you. They are an easy way to conceal problem areas, as well as providing a degree of protection from the sun.

643 DON'T FORGET THE SUPPORT

Swimsuit shopping requires dedication as you'll need to try on lots of different shapes and styles. If you have a bosom that needs support, look for a medium-weight fabric that has a high level of stretch, as well as hidden cups to lift and separate your boobs.

644 ASSESS YOURSELF HONESTLY

Bodies change over the years, and your favourite holiday clothes may no longer be appropriate. Stand in an unforgiving light to try on your beach clothes. It may be time to ditch the bikini in favour of a well-cut swimsuit, which can highlight a great cleavage and hold in a wobbly tummy.

645 WEDDING BELLES

One long-standing rule is that neither the mother of the bride nor the mother of the groom should wear a shade that closely resembles the bride's. The key is to be tasteful and dignified, but never frumpy. Choose a simple luxurious suit or sheath and steer clear of anything flashy, shiny, skimpy, printed or brightly coloured.

646 SECOND-TIME AROUND

The old rules about not wearing white to get remarried no longer apply, and you can choose to wear almost any colour or style of outfit you like the second time around. As a mature bride, you should be aiming for tailored elegance, such as a Jackie Onassis style of matching dress and coat. Avoid an outfit that is too revealing, or anything severely formal and straight-laced, which will look old and frumpy.

jewellery

647 DON'T BE AFRAID OF THE PEARLS

A single string of small pearls and minuscule pearl stud earrings will always have an ageing dowager and somewhat regal look about them. If you like pearls but feel old wearing them, try several strings all at once, like Coco Chanel, or find expensive fakes with larger, chunky-sized stones, which look more modern. Pearls are brilliant for making skin appear more luminescent.

648 CHOKER CRISIS

Women over a certain age should avoid wearing delicate chokers, as they will only draw attention to the neck area. Instead, choose a pendant necklace that forms a V-shape and draws the eye upwards.

649 CHEAP ROCKS

Many chainstores have a great selection of funky and affordable jewellery that can instantly update a look, add a splash of colour and provide a youthful, contemporary touch to an otherwise classic outfit.

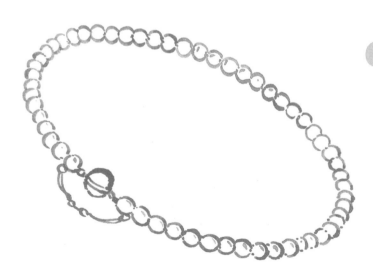

650 STATEMENT JEWELLERY

Quick-fix trinkets can update your look instantly provided you know what's in fashion. A couple of strands of chunky beads will make an ordinary outfit more current if you get the details of size, shape and length right.

651 WATCH THE BREAST LINE

If you feel uncomfortable because of the size of your boobs, don't draw attention to them by wearing a large necklace that nestles right in the centre of your cleavage or, worse still, gets caught around one breast and constantly needs unhooking and re-positioning.

652 BIG DROPPERS SLIM THE FACE

A double chin or round chubby face will benefit from long drop earrings to give the illusion of length. Don't wear heavy earrings for long periods, though, as older skin loses elasticity and ear lobes will get stretched.

653 SIZE MATTERS

The right size of jewellery can help to camouflage figure faults. If you have a short thick neck, avoid tight choker-style necklaces and opt instead for a pendant necklace (not too dainty) that hangs down from your throat, and wear it with a V-neck. If you have a less-than-pert bustline, avoid rounded necklines with circle necklaces, as the line they create repeats the line of the breast, drawing attention to it.

654 CHOOSE VINTAGE OVER BLING

Browse through antique markets for vintage jewellery, which will add personality to everything you wear. Look at fashion magazines to see how to wear your pieces: a brooch or fabric flower pinned to the lapel of a coat will make a big difference.

accessories

655 LONG SCARF TRICKS

If you have a large tummy and want to disguise it, wear a fitted jacket open, keeping the buttons parallel, and then wear a long scarf hanging in between, which will draw attention away from what's hiding underneath.

656 PARISIAN CHIC

Stylish French women know that however beautifully made up your face, a saggy wrinkled neck will always give away your age. Learn how to keep it covered up with a silk scarf tied in a variety of clever styles.

657 THE BEST DISGUISE

Always carry sunglasses in your handbag, even in winter. Low-level winter sun can cause squinting, and sunglasses are the best disguise for tired puffy eyes.

658 WAIST CINCHERS

If you have a tiny waist, show it off with a wide belt. A low-slung belt that cuts across the hips can disguise a bulging tummy.

659 LOOK LIKE AUDREY

Cover up mottled arms with long black evening gloves, just like Audrey Hepburn in *Breakfast at Tiffany's*. Choose Lycra over cotton, as it will provide some support, and wear your biggest rings over the top.

660 DECORATIVE BUCKLES

A studded belt with a highly decorative buckle will attract the eye, but always consider where to place it for maximum effect. Unless you have washboard abs, choose hip-slung, as a belt around the middle tends to cut you in half and shorten the body. A decorative belt replaces the need for long necklaces.

661 BAG A NEW BAG

There's no need to fully update your wardrobe for every new season when one key on-trend item like a fashionable handbag can do it for you. Send your old-lady designer bags to the nearest vintage shop for a twentysomething to make use of – for anyone too much older, they will just look like you're living in the past.

662 ONE SIZE DOESN'T FIT ALL

Collect different handbags for different occasions in your life – one all-purpose black leather handbag stuffed full will wreck your outfit and your posture. For evenings, look for smaller-sized bags made from unusual fabrics and colours that are softer and less structured than your day bag, and do not be tempted to overstuff them and ruin the shape.

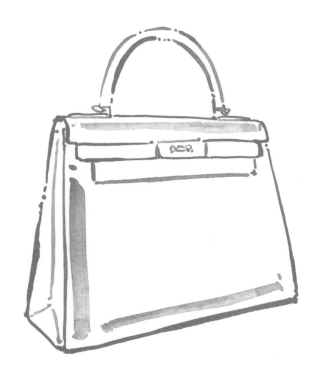

basic fitness principles

663 MAINTAINING GOOD HEALTH

It's a sad fact that with every decade that passes, metabolic rate drops and fat-burning muscles reduce. If you find it easy to put on weight, look seriously at your food and exercise regime. To maintain the same body weight and shape, you will have to exercise more and eat slightly smaller portions. It's worth remembering that 500 g (1 lb) of fat is the equivalent of 3500 calories.

664 TIGHTEN UP 'DOWNSTAIRS'

After childbirth or the menopause, you may find your pelvic floor muscles are not quite up to the job, and that you sometimes experience an embarrassing little leakage when you cough, laugh or go jogging. You can tighten the muscles, either by sucking in and tensing up, as if you were trying to hold a stream of urine, or with a clever device called the Pelvic Toner.

665 EXERCISE FOR BRAIN HEALTH

Moderate exercise can help prevent the slowing down of processes that come with age. It enhances blood flow to the brain, which can reduce the risk of stroke, improves cognitive processing and slows down the degeneration of the nervous system. Don't think of exercise as a short-term punishment that you have to 'put up with'. Make it a part of your daily routine and, after a couple of weeks, it will become second nature to you. Establishing a good habit when you are younger will help you continue with it throughout your senior years.

666 BUILD UP HIGH

Many useful hormones in the body that help maintain energy levels and metabolic rate and control healthy body function can be boosted by moderate exercise. Exercise acts as a major stimulus for the natural secretion of human growth hormone (hGH) and some studies have found that increased hGH, testosterone and endorphins can increase longevity and help to reverse the ageing process.

667 LOSE A LITTLE FOR BIG BENEFITS

If you are overweight, you only have to shed a few pounds to see massive health benefits. Losing just 5–10% of your body weight will lower blood pressure, reduce your risk of diabetes and heart disease, and lower your intake of bad cholesterol. There is also evidence that lower weight corresponds to greater longevity. Losing body fat and creating lean muscles will also improve your overall body shape, while extra muscle will give you a better posture and more energy.

668 LIVE LONG AND WELL

According to a recent study in the *American Journal of Sports Medicine*, the 'greatest threat to health is not the ageing process itself but inactivity'. Moderate physical exercise has been proven to delay the effects of ageing, even if you only start doing it later in life, and possibly increase longevity. The study clearly demonstrated that regular vigorous exercise of just 30 minutes a day is associated with increased life expectancy. Several other studies have shown that colon cancer is reduced by 30% in individuals who exercise regularly.

668 GO FOR THE BURN

For exercise to be beneficial, you need to increase your heart rate, which will improve circulation and metabolism. Sweating is also good, as it encourages the production of sebum, which acts as the skin's own natural moisturizer.

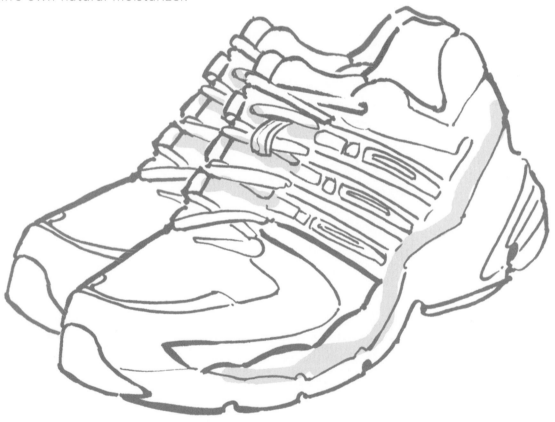

aerobic exercise

670 HIT THE DANCE FLOOR

You're never too old to make a statement on the dance floor; it's good exercise to keep the body loose. Dancing will bring a youthful flush to the cheeks that is only achieved by running 5 km (3 miles) or having great sex.

671 A QUICK STEP TO FITNESS

The simple act of walking will bring significant benefits to your heart and weight. A brisk walk that raises the metabolic rate and makes you a little short of breath will also bring a fresh rosy glow to your cheeks. Buy a clip-on pedometer that can measure your body fat, and aim to walk 10,000 steps a day.

672 UGLY VEINS NEED A SHAKE UP

About 40% of women suffer from ugly varicose veins. Regular aerobic exercise several times a week will get the muscles working and blood pumping through the tiny valves to make the condition much less noticeable.

673 FIGHT CELLULITE WITH FITNESS

Few women athletes have cellulite, as exercise replaces body fat with muscle, and prevents fat cells from becoming blocked with toxins. Jogging, swimming, cycling and walking are all excellent ways to improve circulation and encourage the elimination of toxins.

674 BE AEROBIC FOR FULL-BODY HEALTH

Aerobic exercise provides an overwhelming number of benefits that help to keep the body functioning as it did when it was younger, including boosting circulation, keeping the heart, arteries and veins healthy, perking up the mood and enhancing brain function, helping you to sleep, improving digestion and immunity, and enhancing your skin and general appearance.

675 STEADY SKIPPING

It's so easy even a child can do it, but skipping is a tough calorie-burning workout that is difficult to sustain for 10 minutes. Try to keep your knees bent at all times, barely lifting your feet off the ground, and flicking the rope over your head.

676 RELIEF FOR BACK PAIN

Most cardio exercises involve moves performed in front of the body like tennis, swimming and boxing. Rowing is a great all-round workout that will relieve muscle fatigue from a tired back and neck, releasing tension and stopping frown lines from forming.

677 BREAK INTO A RUN

Walking is good for you but jogging is even better. If you've never jogged a step, then start with walking and jogging – five minutes each for 30 minutes total. Gradually increase the ratio of jogging to walking until it becomes the total exercise time.

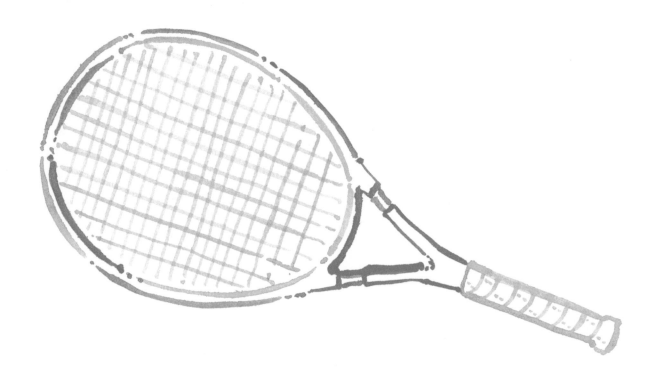

678 GET ON YOUR BIKE

Despite what you may think, cyclists absorb lower levels of pollutants from traffic fumes than car drivers, and research has shown that if you cycle regularly, you can expect to be as fit as an average person 10 years younger.

679 BOUNCE AWAY PAIN

Mini rebounders that fit inside your bedroom provide a great aerobic workout for all levels of fitness and ages, though older people will need to do gentler, less gymnastic moves. Rebounding protects joints from hard-impact exercise and offers relief from neck and back pains. It also strengthens leg muscles and increases oxygen availability throughout the body.

680 NO WATER NEEDED

The advantage of a rowing machine is that it offers an all-over workout with very little impact on joints. Vigorous rowing is one of the most effective calorie-burning exercises, but you can set your own pace, and it will tone up flabby arms and help give you a flatter stomach.

681 WORK IT!

To make your cardiovascular training effective, you should be prepared to work out at least 3–5 days a week for a duration of about 20 minutes. Incorporate interval training into your workout so you include 'light' exercise with 'hard' work, where you intensify the heartbeat to 70–100% of the maximum heart rate.

682 SMASHING SQUASH

Bashing a tiny rubber ball around a court has to be one of the most energetic things you can do with a friend or on your own. The smashing action is a great stressbuster, and a 30-minute game of squash will leave you with better aerobic fitness, as well as toning and strengthening all muscle groups.

683 CLIMB EVERY MOUNTAIN

If you're going out for a weekend walk, choose a route with as many hills as possible. This will be a better workout for your heart and have a greater toning effect on the wobbly bits, particularly the calves, thighs and bottom.

684 JUMP IN

Swimming is one of the most effective fat-burning exercises you can do, as you are simultaneously working both the upper and lower body against the water. It is great for toning flabby arms and legs, and is achievable regardless of your overall level of fitness.

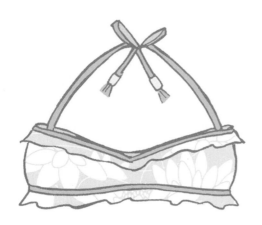

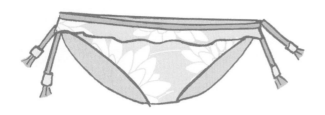

weight & resistance training

685 INCREASE YOUR METABOLISM

Strength-training exercises can raise the metabolic rate by about 30–50 calories per day. Over a three-month period, appropriate training will produce about 1.4 kg (3 lb) of muscle, which will boost your resting metabolic rate by about 7%.

686 WEIGHT TRAIN FOR BONE STRENGTH

Using free weights a couple of times a week for all-over strength training will significantly increase bone-mineral density in the spine, helping to stop vertebrae collapsing and decreasing your chances of losing height.

687 GRAB A SET OF FREE WEIGHTS

Research has shown that free weights are more effective at building muscle tone than pushing against the resistance of machine weights. Plus you can use them at home or anywhere, any time.

688 PUMP IT UP

Pumping iron of any kind increases your metabolism for the time of the workout and for a few hours afterwards. What's more, it will help you convert body fat to lean muscle. Not only does this look great, but muscle burns more calories than fat, so it's a double whammy!

689 BUILD MUSCLE TO BURN CALORIES

Muscle burns up to three times as many calories as any other tissue, and is the most metabolically active part of your body. Add some resistance training to your routine to help you burn off calories in your downtime and shape up even after you've finished working out.

690 SIZE DOES MATTER

If weights are small, you might just as well be lifting a pencil above your head. Even if you don't want to 'build' muscle, you need to create overload to cause the muscle to get firmer and stronger, so push yourself to use a free weight that will challenge you.

691 BEEF UP YOUR BONES

Hormonal changes and poor nutrition can cause bones to get thinner as we age. Incorporating resistance weight training into your weekly routine will help maintain bone density and ward off osteoporosis.

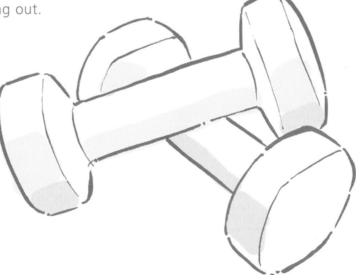

155

682 INCREASE ENERGY EXPENDITURE

As well as burning energy while you work out, a study from the American College of Sports Medicine found that the metabolic rate remained elevated for two hours after strength-training with weights – burning off more calories while you do nothing.

693 STRENGTHEN MUSCLES TO HELP YOUR BONES

Osteoporosis is a main cause of disability in women as they age, particularly post-menopause, but don't let fear of breaking bones stop you from the one thing that can help – exercise. More muscle will help support your skeletal structure and will help you retain good balance and posture, which in turn will help you avoid falls.

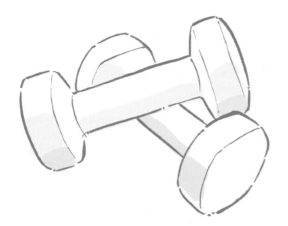

flexibility exercises

684 PRACTISE STATIC FLEXIBILITY

Static-active flexibility describes a movement that uses only your own muscle group to extend a position; for example, lifting a leg and holding it in position. Static-passive describes a movement that requires other forces to maintain the position, such as a chair or your own body weight. Aim to incorporate both types in your workout for maximum benefit.

695 WAKE UP THE FEEL-GOOD CHEMICALS

Work up a sweat in just 10 minutes with some serious stretching and eight sun salutations every morning when you get out of bed. It will boost the mood-enhancing chemicals dopamine, norepinephrine and serotonin.

696 STRETCH FOR GOOD POSTURE

When your joints are stiff, your abdominal and chest muscles become tight, pulling you forwards into a stooped position. Chest and shoulder stretches, as well as push-ups, will counter these effects.

697 TOUCH YOUR TOES FOR ENERGY

For a quick shot of energy when you need it, bend over at the waist and hang your head down so that your hands touch your toes (or as near as you can get), and you're looking at your knees. Relax your upper body. Hold the position for several seconds and then slowly rise. This is a good morning starter that will also increase flexibility and help you align your posture.

698 INCREASE YOUR RANGE OF MOTION

Your stretch routine should address each section of the body and be dynamic, which means bringing a limb or muscle group through its full range of motion slowly and smoothly.

699 HALT THE SHRINKING PROCESS

A strong straight back is key to keeping the height you had at 20. After the age of 40, we shrink 1 cm ($\frac{1}{2}$ inch) every 10 years, so practise lying on your tummy with arms outstretched in front of you, and gently raise one arm for the count of 10 as you breathe out. Repeat 8 times with both arms.

700 INCREASE YOUR MOBILITY

Your joints can tighten and become thicker as you age but flexibility exercises can help increase the mobility. Bending, rotating and extending your joints prevents injury, so follow a good gentle stretching regime four or five days a week. Avoid any positions that can compress your vertebrae and put undue stress on your spine, however, such as vigorous forward or side twists.

701 EASY DOES IT

Stretching is a gentle, easy exercise, so don't approach it as if you were racing through your workout. Be patient, use slow, deep movements and never force it so you feel pain. Take your time and breathe naturally during your stretch, taking care never to hold your breath. If any stretch hurts you, eliminate it from your routine.

beating middle-aged spread

702 SORT OUT THE SOMATOPAUSE

Medical practitioners have defined the onset of middle-aged spread as the somatopause. Strenuous aerobic exercise has been shown to increase the production of hGH (the human growth hormone that is responsible for this metabolic slow-down), helping to reverse classic middle-aged symptoms.

703 IT'S CRUNCH TIME

Abdominal crunches are the best way to tone all the muscle groups of the stomach, so make sure you don't neglect them. Regular exercises will strengthen the core muscle groups of the trunk, where all your body's movements originate. These muscles support your internal organs, aid in breathing and work with the vertebrae to help your body bend and twist.

704 TUMMY TIGHTENER

Most of us spend far too many hours at work but when you are sitting at your desk, focus on tightening your tummy and your bottom, hold for 20 seconds, then relax for 20. Do this four times a day and you will notice the difference.

705 WAIST AWAY FOR OPTIMUM HEALTH

People prone to the 'apple' shape and with a waist measurement of over 81 cm (32 in) need to act now to avert the potential danger of heart disease and diabetes. Losing even a small amount of weight, 10% of your body weight, will drastically reduce this dangerous layer of tummy fat by 30%.

706 TONE THAT TUMMY

Shape up effortlessly with a Slendertone corset that stimulates muscles in the abdomen without you having to do a thing. Small pulsing contractions train muscles to be firmer and stronger, and regular use will reduce the size of the waist.

707 TOP TUMMY TIP

Strengthen your core and build arm muscles by resting your tummy on an exercise ball and then walking on your hands as far as you can so that the ball slowly moves towards your feet. Keep your body as straight as possible, then walk backwards.

708 TIGHTEN UP THE TORSO

Rollerblading and ice-skating are both good for keeping the torso strong and toned. The arms propel motion, while the upper body has to stay strong to provide balance, working all the abdomen muscles in the process.

709 BUM AND TUM LIFT

If you need a rest, this exercise involves lying flat on your back. Rest your ankles on an exercise ball, then slowly raise your hips so that your body is in a straight line from the shoulders to the ankles. Hold for 30 seconds, then lower your hips. Repeat 10 times.

710 TONE THE TRUNK WITH PILATES

In middle age, the build-up of fat from a reduced metabolism usually forms around the waist and stomach. Pilates lessons focus on core stability exercises that target this trunk area to tone up the waist and stomach, as well as strengthening the lumbar region of the spine.

711 SIT UP AND WORK OUT

Just sitting on an exercise ball in front of the TV will provide benefits. Sit up straight, tighten your tummy muscles and gently lift one foot off the floor at a time. Do this while watching your favourite programme – multitasking is what we're good at!

712 DON'T LOVE YOUR LOVE HANDLES

Waist twists will help you target those unsightly love handles. It is a very low-impact exercise and a good precursor to abdominal crunch work. Stand with your feet flat on the floor, your fingertips touching the tops of your shoulders, and your arms bent at the elbow. Slowly twist the elbows, arms and shoulder, as if you are looking over your shoulder, following the movement of your upper body with your head, and keep your abdominal muscles tensed. Rotate to the other side.

bottoms & legs

713 IN-LINE FOR A PERT BOTTOM

For a workout that targets the backs of the thighs and the bottom more effectively than running or cycling, try 30 minutes of in-line skating. It works the hip muscles and tightens up the gluteus maximus without too much hard work.

714 ANY TIME, ANY PLACE

Waiting at the bus stop or in the checkout queue at the supermarket can be time well spent if you clench your bottom and hold it for 30 seconds at a time. This will work the gluteus maximus muscles to firm up a flabby bottom and protect the lower spine.

715 TARGET THE INNER THIGH

Thighs that jiggle do not have to be a fact of life. Your hip adductors are those small muscles on the inner thighs that help you pull your legs together and apart. The most effective exercises for toning this area rely on the use of weights, bands or balls to provide resistance. Side-stepping squats and lunges are also effective.

716 A BETTER BOTTOM

You probably can't change your natural body shape but you can tighten up a flabby derrière with regular lunging exercises. Stand up straight, take a big step forward and bend at the knee, then push back up to a standing position.

717 THE BEST BOTTOM CLENCH

To keep your butt fit and taut, get in the habit of performing an easy leg lift every time you clean your teeth. Hold onto the basin and lift one leg out to the side and back, keeping the movement slow and controlled with the foot flexed.

718 INCREASING SINGLE-LEG STRENGTH

Exercises to tone all the muscle groups of the legs will keep you in good stead and allow you to maintain shapely pins. However, most exercises use conventional double-leg training, which isn't as effective as developing single-leg strength. Working one leg at a time independently will help you with all your leg transitions – when you move from one leg to another, which is when you walk, run, step, reach or lunge.

719 SLIM THE SADDLEBAGS

To target the outer thigh area, which is prone to unsightly lumps known as 'saddlebags', stand up straight and lift your right leg out to the side and then lower it. Remain erect without leaning, and repeat 10–12 times, before repeating with the other leg. For a more intensive workout, strap on light ankle-weights.

720 LEG LUNGES FOR SHAPELY KNEES

If your knees are showing their age with crepey loose skin above the kneecap, try incorporating leg lunges and squats into your workout routine. Leg muscles build up quickly in just a few weeks, and the lunges target the quad muscles at the front of the thigh, which support the knee. The hamstrings and glutes will also get a good workout.

attack bingo wings

721 SHOP AND TONE

When you're at the supermarket, forget the shopping trolley and use a basket instead. This will help tone your arms, particularly if you do a few biceps curls while standing in the checkout queue!

722 WEIGHTS MAKE A DIFFERENCE

Make your power walk even more effective by carrying small hand weights with you. Walk purposefully, using your arms to move you along. Exercising in this way will benefit your arms and legs simultaneously.

723 WORK OUT WITH WEIGHTS

Cardiovascular work isn't enough to keep muscle tone built up as we get older. Regular arm exercises that use the same muscles repeatedly will result in beautifully contoured arms, and a faster metabolism, as muscle burns more calories than fat.

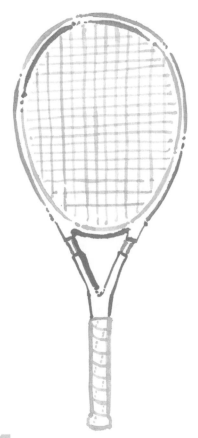

725 EVERYDAY ARM DIPS

No one wants bingo wings, as they are the surest sign of middle age. To make sure your upper arms are never an embarrassment, do triceps dips whenever you can – all you need is a chair!

726 BIG BALL PRESS-UPS

You will need to concentrate to stop yourself from falling off when you start doing press-ups (push-ups) on an exercise ball, but this manoeuvre will make a big difference. Three sets of 10, three times a week, are all you need to reduce flabby bingo wings and tone up core muscles.

737 INTELLECTUAL WORKOUT

Another at-home exercise for your arms that will keep muscle tone firm and smooth is to clasp a heavy book in each hand then do arm lifts, from resting at your side to reaching out to shoulder level. While you've still got that heavy book in your hands, try lying flat on your back with your arms outstretched above your head. Now raise your arms until the book is above your head – try three sets of 10, three times a week.

734 PLAY TENNIS FOR TRICEPS TONING

The triceps muscles at the back of the arms make up two-thirds of the arm's size so strengthening this hard-to-reach area will make a noticeable improvement to your arms' shape. Practising your overhead swing can really help with toning, as can triceps dips and kickbacks.

ancient arts

728 HOLD DOWNWARD DOG

Take a yoga lesson to bring together the body, mind and spirit into an integrated whole. The physical benefits are increased flexibility, strength and stamina, as well as an inner sense of wellbeing, positivity and clarity.

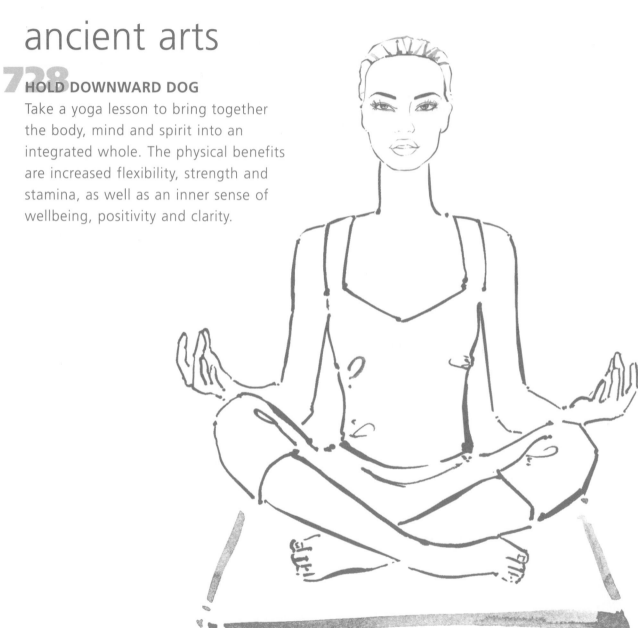

729 STAND ON YOUR HEAD

Get into the habit of standing on your head first thing in the morning. In yoga, this pose is called the 'king of asanas' because of the rejuvenating effect it has on just about every cell in the body. It is thought to slow down the ageing process dramatically.

730 STRENGTHEN YOUR SPINE

The shoulderstand is a challenging yoga pose that has great benefits for the whole body. It's important to warm up before going into it, but it boosts circulation, stimulates the thyroid gland and strengthens the shoulders, arms and upper back.

731 MEDITATION IN MOTION

The ancient Chinese art of t'ai chi is a non-competitive type of exercise that has physical as well as mental benefits. It is used to reduce stress, and increase energy and general feelings of wellbeing.

good posture

732 AVOID OLD-AGE SLUMP

When meeting new people, be aware of standing upright and tucking your bottom in. Avoid slouching, slumping and leaning against walls to prop yourself up. Take your hands out of your pockets, and straighten rounded shoulders. Nothing is more ageing than a hunched back and poor posture.

733 I MUST, I MUST, IMPROVE MY BUST

Improved posture can create the illusion of a bigger chest. Make a conscious effort to stand up straight, as an erect spine naturally lifts the ribcage and enables the breasts to sit more pertly on the chest. Seek assistance from a chiropractor if you can't improve your posture on your own.

734 RELAX YOUR SHOULDERS

Tension, stress and anxiety all make us scrunch our shoulders up, giving us the appearance of a hunchback, as well as head and neck ache. Remind yourself to push your shoulders back and down, and relax the muscles for better posture.

735 CHOOSE AN ERGONOMIC CHAIR

Sitting in an ergonomically designed chair while you work will reduce the damage of hunched shoulders and a bad back, but you should still have a regular spinal stretch and roll your head from side to side to help keep your back straight and strong.

736 SIT PRETTY TO AVOID NECK PAIN

Common causes of neck pain are the natural degeneration of the spine and poor posture. Prevent pain by maintaining a good posture when you are sitting for long periods. Avoid performing tasks that can strain the neck, such as reading or knitting, for prolonged periods. Change your position periodically, and avoid napping in chairs, as the neck can cramp uncomfortably.

737 GAIN HEIGHT WITH PILATES

Pilates exercises help maintain a straight, strong spine, and keeping the spine aligned correctly in a controlled way will help prevent the spine from curving. To stay in alignment, imagine a piece of string that runs vertically through your spine and pulls your head upwards.

738 WALK TALL THE ALEXANDER WAY

Good posture is one of the best and easiest ways to defy age. The Alexander Technique teaches you to stand, sit and walk in perfect alignment. It also improves stamina and flexibility.

choosing fitness clothing

739 HARDER-WORKING TRAINERS

The Power Diet sports shoe is the latest high-achieving trainer. It is available with two sets of ergonomically designed, weighted insoles to make your muscles work harder as you run. It is especially effective for toning flabby legs.

740 AVOID ACHILLES INJURY

Only wear your running shoes for running, as playing other sports in them will significantly break down their motion control and cushioning. Replace them every six months, as the cushioning designed to protect your feet does wear out.

741 PROTECT YOUR BOOBS

Breasts need to be held firmly in position when you exercise or they will bounce around and cause stretching of the Coopers ligament, which is the only ligament that stops the breast from sagging. Once stretched, it is irreversible, and you will be left with saggy bosoms forever.

742 MAKE THE MOST OF YOUR MBT TRAINERS

Search out the latest high-tech footwear that will maximize your workout when you wear them. By transforming hard and artificial surfaces into natural and uneven ground, every step taken in Masai Barefoot Technology trainers becomes more of a workout, toning and shaping the body and encouraging perfect posture.

743 CHOOSE FASHIONABLE KIT

Exercise clothes don't have to be shapeless grey sweatpants, which will only make you look and feel older than you are. Find clothes you feel comfortable in and that flatter you; if you think you look like a fat elephant every time you get ready to go for a work out, you will feel depressed and demoralized and make excuses not to go.

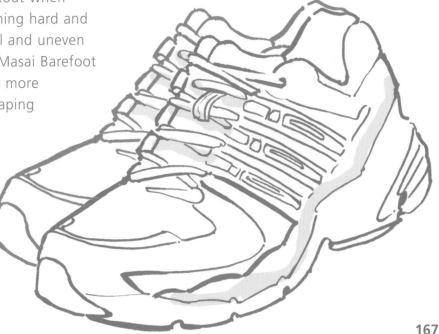

fitting fitness into everyday life

744 SUPPORT YOUR TEAM

If your children play for a football (soccer) team, volunteer to be a 'linesman'. Running up and down the touchline for an hour is great exercise, and because you'll be cheering them on at the same time, you won't even notice how much running you're doing. Take every opportunity you have to exercise with your kids – not only will it help your health but you will also become a role model for them and help them establish good healthy habits.

745 FORGET TO SIT DOWN

Try to do your ordinary tasks while standing or walking around, as this will help you avoid spending long periods of time sitting, which can lead to an increased risk of thrombosis and swollen ankles. For example, every time the phone rings, stand up and walk around to talk.

746 DON'T LIKE THE GYM – DON'T GO!

If you find the treadmill boring, find some other aerobic exercise that is fun and challenging. Tennis, salsa dancing, fencing or ballet will all increase your heartbeat, keeping you fit and supple, and they are also good social opportunities.

747 THE JOY OF BIKES

Rediscover the pleasure of cycling to and from the shops. Short hops will tone up legs and calves, and if you really start to enjoy it, you can start muddy mountain biking, which will improve all-over fitness and bring a rosy glow to your skin.

748 HANG IT HIGH

If you hang your washing outside on the line, make sure the line is high above your head. Endless reaching up to peg the clothes will give your spine a thorough stretch and stop you hunching. Make the most of other chores around the house, too, such as getting a good upper-body workout from washing your car or vigorous spring cleaning.

748 KEEP MOVING

Every day think of something you can do to get the blood pumping. Always take the most energetic option if you have a choice: walk up stairs instead of taking the lift (elevator), and even walk up escalators if you can. Take a bike ride instead of using the car for short distances, or park the car some distance away from your destination and walk the rest of the way.

750 WORK IT OUT

Get outside in the garden and do some physical digging, raking or shovelling soil. Research has shown that an afternoon spent gardening uses as much energy as casual cycling or walking, and the whole body gets a workout, as you are lifting, stretching and occasionally weightlifting.

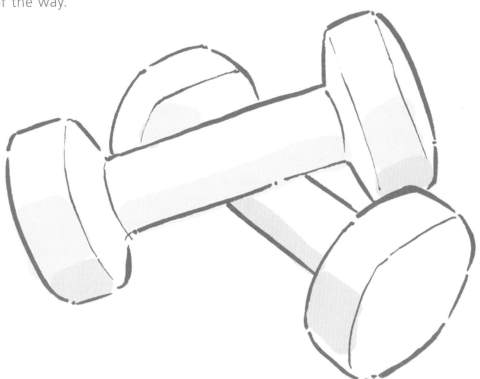

antiageing superfoods

751 CHECK OUT ORAC FOODS

Oxygen Radical Absorbance Capacity (ORAC) is an American test-tube analysis that has pinpointed the highest levels of antioxidants in fruit and vegetables. Early findings by the US Department of Agriculture suggest ORAC foods may help slow the ageing process in the brain as well as the body, and young and middle-aged people may be able to reduce the risk of diseases of ageing, including senility, by eating high-ORAC foods.

752 TOP-SCORING ORAC FOODS

The high levels of antioxidants found in the ORAC foods (see above) come from plant pigments called polyphenols, and it is thought to be the combination of vitamins, iron and folic acid that makes them so effective. Top-scoring ORAC foods are avocado, blueberries, broccoli, garlic, kale, plums, raisins, red grapes and spinach.

753 A GOOD CUPPA TEA

Repeated exposure to a daily dose of pollution, stress, cigarette smoke and sunlight ensures we all have to cope with more than 10 million free radical hits a day. Drinking a daily mug of green or white tea can promote antioxidant activity and lower chances of free radical problems. It has also been claimed that if you dunk the teabag up and down in the water it releases more of its antioxidant properties.

754 FEED THE INSIDE FOR RESULTS ON THE OUTSIDE

Make sure your diet includes plenty of antioxidants, which are found in abundance in fresh fruit and vegetables. These will help to slow down cellular ageing, and also work to 'disarm' the body's bad cells.

755 BE AN OLD PRUNE

Dried plums – prunes – have been given the ultimate superfood status, as they are thought to contain the highest level of antioxidants, which neutralize the dangerous free radicals associated with DNA degradation and accelerated ageing.

756 COOK UP PERFECT SKIN

If you want skin that's as smooth as a tomato, then eat one! Tomatoes contain lycopene, a skin-friendly antioxidant that is also thought to reduce the risk of cancer. Cooking tomatoes makes lycopene more readily absorbable by the body, so choose tomato sauces over the raw fruits in salads.

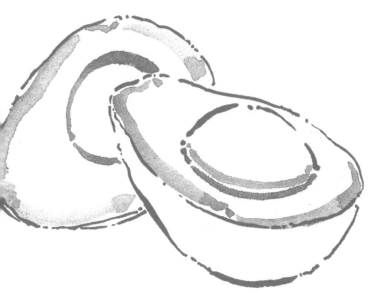

757 THE POWERS OF 'A'

Vitamin A is a true wonder vitamin. Not only can it soothe and rejuvenate the skin, but it may actually be able to prevent sun damage. Liver, sweet potato, carrots, mangoes, spinach and milk are all great sources.

758 FULL-FAT SKINCARE

A diet that is devoid of all fats will deprive your skin of the essential fatty acids it needs, and leave your skin looking dry and dull. Essential Fatty Acids (EFAs) are absolutely vital for good health, as they help lower cholesterol and keep hair and skin healthy. They can't be made in your body so they must be supplied through your diet. Nuts, avocado and oily fish are all good sources.

759 ZINC IT UP

When it comes to skin-boosting minerals, zinc is the first choice, as it has a direct effect on the regeneration of skin from the inside out, which can help ageing and problem skins. Zinc is mostly found in protein-based foods but vegetarians can find a great source in pumpkin seeds.

760 SPECIFIC HEALTH BOOSTERS

Purple anthocyanins that are found in blueberries are known to strengthen tiny blood vessels and so help reduce spider veins and the flushed red appearance of rosacea.

761 STAY CALM

The most useful of vitamins for healthy skin, vitamin A has the ability to calm red and blotchy skin and is also thought to visibly reduce lines and wrinkles.

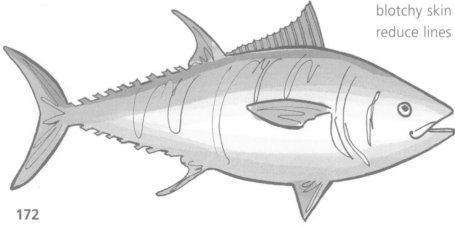

762 SARDINES FOR SUPPER

It is recommended that women eat two portions of oily fish a week, and sardines provide an easy way to achieve this – served on toast, they make a perfect early-evening snack. High in omega-3 fatty acids, they provide some of the best protection against heart disease and strokes, and help to keep skin soft, supple and young-looking.

763 BRILLIANT BEER

Traditionally, beer has always been thought to be good for the hair and the skin. Now we know it is rich in silic acid, the dissolved version of the trace mineral silicon, which is found in the skin, so beer is officially good for you.

764 LOOK FOR NUTRACEUTICALS

Wise up to 'functional foods' that have specific health benefits because they have had health-boosting extras added to them, like margarine spread that has plant sterols to help lower cholesterol, or water with added calcium.

765 CHEER UP WITH CHERRIES

For a quick burst of something sweet that will give you instant energy and raise blood sugar levels slowly, eat cherries. They contain antioxidants called flavonoids, which have been reported to have antiviral, anti-allergic, antiplatelet, anti-inflammatory, antitumour and antioxidant activities.

766 SWEET AS HONEY

Renowned for its medicinal properties since the time of the ancient Egyptians, dark-coloured honeys such as buckwheat possess more antioxidants than the lighter varieties, and also provide nutrients for the growth of new tissue, helping skin rejuvenate itself and stay young-looking.

767 EAT YOUR GREENS

Learn to love green foods like cabbage, leeks and broccoli, which are rich in sulphur, the 'beauty mineral' that promotes healthy skin and nails. They also contain high levels of antioxidants, which help to prevent skin from ageing.

768 GO GREEN

Ditch sweet milky tea in favour of healthy herbal teas without milk and sugar; there are lots of varieties to choose from. As well as being full of antioxidants, green tea is thought to speed up calorie burning.

769 SEARCH OUT SELENIUM

This is a very important antioxidant that works with vitamin E to prohibit free-radical damage to the cell membrane. It is also thought to help prevent cancer, protect against heart and circulatory diseases and promote healthy eyes, skin and hair. Good natural sources include Brazil nuts, kidney, liver and wholemeal bread.

770 DO ORGANIC DAIRY

Recent research has shown that organic dairy products are much better for us than non-organic. They contain higher levels of vitamin E, omega-3 fatty acids and antioxidants, all of which have positive antiageing properties.

771 SELENIUM-RICH FOODS

Products that have been grown in selenium-enriched soil (wheat for bread, and potatoes) can help to provide the body's ideal intake of selenium, which contains a powerful antioxidant, strenghtens the immune system and helps maintain a strong heart.

772 BE A CHOCOHOLIC

Flavonoids are super nutrients that help protect the body from potentially dangerous free radical cells. They are found in good-quality dark chocolate that contains at least 70% cocoa solids.

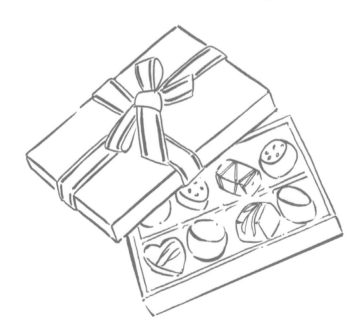

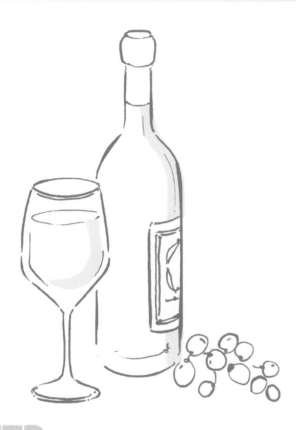

774 NUTTY ABOUT NUTS

Unsalted nuts make a great snack, as they are full of EFAs, which can't be manufactured by the body and which are needed to speed up the digestive system and keep skin moist and fresh-looking. Stick to a small handful because they are highly calorific.

775 ONE AMAZING LITTLE BERRY

Known as one of the antiageing super foods, the acai berry is indigenous to the Amazon rainforests, and contains the same compounds called anthocyanins that make red wine good for us. Try concentrated fruit drinks, or eat the berry itself, to help slow down the ageing process.

773 RED WINE EVERY TIME

A natural compound called resveratrol, which is found in the skin of grapes and is present in red wine, is a powerful antioxidant that may protect against cancer and cardiovascular disease, as well as helping the body to break down fat.

776 STRONG COLOURS COUNT MORE

All fresh fruit and vegetables contain powerful antioxidants but, in general, the deeper and more intense the colour, the higher the content. Choose red and orange pepper, tomatoes, cranberries, pomegranates and broccoli.

777 A SHOT OF WHEATGRASS

It may taste unusual, but a small glass of wheatgrass is packed with many essential minerals including calcium, magnesium, potassium, iron and sodium as well as vitamins A, B C and E, all of which are needed for healthy teeth, hair and skin. It's very easy to grow your own.

778 HEALTHY INSIDE AND OUT

Low-fat organic yogurt is not only rich in vitamin A, which is needed to boost cell regeneration, but also contains acidophilus, the 'live ' bacteria that is good for the gut. A boost of vitamin A, accompanied by a healthy digestive system, is going to be reflected in a fabulous skin tone.

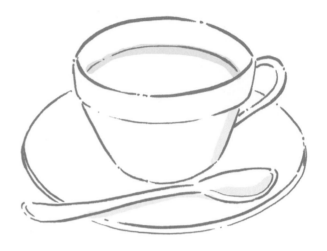

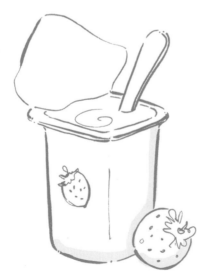

779 BUSH BENEFITS

Try bush tea instead of the traditional cuppa. A herbal brew drunk for centuries by the San of southern Africa, its taste is similar to ordinary tea. It's also caffeine-free and packed with antioxidants.

780 GOJI GOOD FOR CELLULITE

One leading skincare expert has dubbed goji juice the 'cellulite assassin'. This energy-boosting drink contains more betacarotene than carrots and more iron than spinach.

781 FROZEN FOOD CAN BE GOOD FOR YOU

Frozen berries are filled with just as many healthy antioxidants as fresh ones, and make an excellent source of vitamin C in winter. They also contain small amounts of vitamin A and calcium.

782 CHEW UP ON ALMOND SKINS

Almond skins contain 20 potent antioxidants to protect against heart disease. They are also rich in vitamin E, which is thought to help slow down the ageing process.

783 DON'T PEEL

Always eat the peel from apples and pears because this is where all the potent antioxidants are found. The peel also provides insoluble fibre that helps to prevent digestive problems.

784 ENERGY-BOOSTING BERRY

Freshly juiced blackcurrants contain a host of antioxidants that can protect cells from premature ageing, as well as lower cholesterol levels and guard against cancer.

785 TYPHOO TEA IS GOOD FOR YOU

Green tea and black tea contain a different amount of polyphenols, but both can help the immune system fight off infection and help skin cell rejuvenation.

786 CRUNCH ON BETACAROTENE

Organic carrots are a great source of betacarotene, a powerful antiageing antioxidant that the body converts into vitamin A, which promotes healthy skin and cells and good night vision.

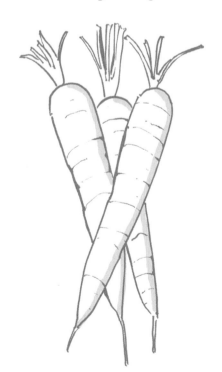

vitamins & supplements

787 REJUVENATE WITH C

This multitasking vitamin reaches every cell in the body. Known as ascorbic acid, it is vital for collagen production and, as a powerful antioxidant, it destroys harmful free radicals that cause premature ageing.

788 KEEP IT BALANCED

A balanced diet should contain all the essential vitamins and minerals we need, as well as essential protein, carbohydrate, fats and fibre. Vitamin supplements should never be relied on to replace good-quality food.

789 COLLAGEN CAPSULES

Beautiful skin comes from within, and collagen capsules contain vital proteins and amino acids that help stimulate the body's own collagen production, giving you firmer, plumper-looking skin.

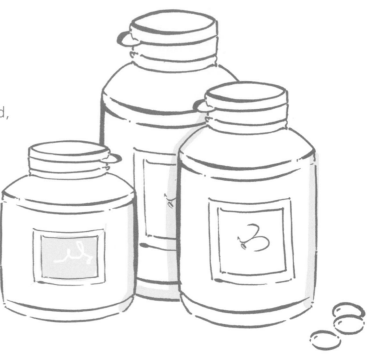

790 NO MAGIC PILLS

If supplements are used merely to counterbalance poor eating habits, the improvements in skin tone, nail growth and hair texture will all be negligible. Overdosing on supplements can do more harm than good, and could make you ill.

781 B WISE WITH BORAGE

Improve overall health with borage oil. Derived from the seeds of borage, it is packed full of GLA (gamma linolenic acid), a 'good' fat that promotes healthy skin, hair and nail growth by supplying the body with essential fatty acids.

782 GO STARRY-EYED WITH COENZYME Q10

This powerful antioxidant and moisturizer is the movie stars' favourite. It occurs naturally in the skin, and can accelerate cell repair. Taken in tablet form, it provides mechanisms for the body to heal itself, so after prolonged use it can rejuvenate the skin as it begins to function better.

783 BEAUTY FROM THE INSIDE

Take a course of Imedeen supplements, which contain biomarine complex, a fish extract that is similar to the proteins found naturally in the skin's supportive tissue. The extract has been proven to improve the density and moisture content of the skin.

784 FLEXI-OIL

If you were given cod liver oil as a child without knowing why, there is now evidence that a capsule a day can reduce pain and inflammation in joints, keeping them flexible and supple, as well as promoting healthy skin, hair and nails.

785 SUPPLEMENTS MAY BOOST PERFORMANCE

As nutrition from food has been compromised by pollution, pesticides and processing, a daily dietary supplement in the form of vitamins, minerals or fish oils may help keep you at the optimum levels of health and fitness.

786 GO FOR GINSENG

The root of this plant, which contains ginsenocide, is used as a tonic to strengthen the immune system, increase concentration, boost energy levels and generally revitalize the whole body.

787 BENEFITS OF POND LIFE

Spirulina is a type of blue-green algae found in most lakes and ponds, and consumed for thousands of years by Mexican Aztecs. It is a very rich source of protein, vitamin B complex, vitamin E and zinc, and is used in many skincare products to promote healthy skin and hair.

788 THE NATURAL PROZAC

The herbal supplement St John's Wort can help ease feelings of depression and lift black moods. It is thought to increase the activity and prolong the action of the neurotransmitters serotonin and noradrenalin in a similar way to standard antidepressants, and will need to be taken for a few weeks before it starts working.

789 POP A PILL

There is no substitute for a healthy diet, but taking a multivitamin every day will ensure you are getting the right vitamins and minerals to maintain an active lifestyle. For best results, take your supplements with meals, as they work synergistically with other nutrients.

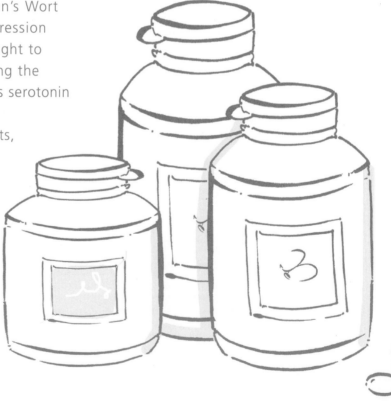

800 REMEMBER REMEMBER

Scientific analysis has found that the chemicals found in ginkgo biloba include flavonoids and terpenoids, which mop up free radicals and reduce blood clotting and inflammation. Devotees believe this extract of the maidenhair tree improves memory and concentration.

801 EAT YOURSELF SMARTER

A brain-boosting supplement such as ginkgo biloba or hawthorn may help to improve mental function, stimulating memory cells, keeping you alert and helping to rejuvenate brain cell activity.

802 SMOOTHER SKIN WITH CENTELLA

First accepted as a drug in France in the 1880s, the extract of this herb has been reintroduced by the cosmetics industry as a treatment for cellulite. It is thought to enhance the connective tissue structure and reduce sclerosis of the fibroblasts, making skin smoother.

803 TAKE A TIME-DEFYING SUPPLEMENT

To help maintain a radiant and more youthful complexion, take Perfectil Platinum. Designed to regenerate and refine ageing skin, its ingredients include high-grade marine collagen, pine bark extract and alpha-lipoic acid.

804 HORSE CHESTNUT BENEFITS

Available in creams, tablets and capsules from health food stores and pharmacies, horse chestnut seeds have long been used as a treatment for varicose veins and haemorrhoids. The horse chestnut contains aescin, which may help reduce the appearance of cellulite by toning the capillaries below the skin.

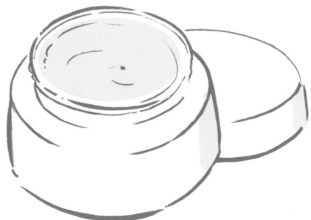

805 OILS TO BEAT THE COLD

The cold winter wind can make skin severely dehydrated, chapped and flaky. To minimize the damage, increase your intake of omega-3 oils by eating more oily fish and taking an omega-3 supplement to keep skin plump and hydrated.

806 BARKING UP THE RIGHT TREE

Pycnogenol describes a class of powerful bioflavonoids that have been extracted from pine tree bark. Pycnogenol protects skin against photo-ageing, and has the ability to revitalize collagen.

807 WARM HANDS

Make sure your hands are warm, as flu viruses and colds often start with cold hands. In winter, bad circulation can be treated with a variety of herbal remedies to warm up the body, such as ginkgo biloba or cayenne. Hawthorn is also well known for helping to keep blood vessels relaxed and allowing a freer flow of blood throughout the body.

808 GET CALM WITH MAGNOLIA

A supplement made from magnolia bark extract has been found to relieve anxiety, calm nerves, ward off stress and boost the metabolism. Taken on a regular basis, it is believed to lift your mood and improve general wellbeing, as well as reduce levels of cortisol (the stress hormone). High cortisol levels can compromise the immune system and lead to loss of vitality, weight gain and high blood pressure.

809 LATE NIGHT REPAIR

As you get older, it takes your body – and your skin – longer to recover from late nights. If you've been out into the small hours instead of sleeping, your skin will have had less time to oxygenate, eliminate waste and repair itself. A superfood supplement like the organic pharmacy phytonutrients based on wheat and barley grasses, and detoxifying chlorella, will feed nutrients back from the inside and let your skin bounce back to health.

illnesses & conditions

810 NATURAL PAINKILLERS

Up your intake of organic fruit and vegetables and you could kiss your aches and pains goodbye. Red fruit like pomegranates are a particularly rich source of antioxidants, which have the ability to neutralize the chemicals in the body that cause long-term pain and inflammation.

811 DRINK PROBIOTIC FOR GOOD DIGESTION

Probiotic drinks are pocket-sized health drinks that introduce good 'bugs' into the digestive system. The live bacteria *Bifidobacterium bifidum* BB-12 combine with the existing good bacteria in the gut and help to get rid of harmful bacteria. They are known to aid digestion and other gut-related problems.

812 MAKE A DATE WITH THE DOCTOR

Knowing and listening to your own body becomes more important as you get older. Get screened for diseases like cancer and heart disease regularly, before little problems turn into unmanageable ones.

813 KEEP LIVER HEALTHY WITH MILK THISTLE

This herb has lasting benefits for the liver. Trials have proved it can prevent and heal damage to this vital organ and that it also has a significant effect on cirrhosis and chronic hepatitis.

814 FIGHT IBS

If you suffer from irritable bowel syndrome (IBS), avoid fizzy drinks, which are loaded with phosphates that deplete the body of vital minerals and interfere with digestion. Fresh water and juices are much better for your digestion.

815 KEEP YOUR COLON HEALTHY

New prebiotic products provide an efficient way to increase friendly bacteria in the bowel. They stimulate the growth of lactic acid bacteria such as *Lactobacillus acidophilus* and may help to reduce the risk of many gastrointestinal illnesses. Prebiotics occur naturally in Jerusalem artichokes, garlic, onions and asparagus.

816 CUT CANCER CHANCES

A diet that contains good quantities of cruciferous vegetables, like broccoli, kale, cabbage, cauliflower and sprouts, is estimated to contribute to a 50% reduction in the incidence of cancerous tumours because they contain isothiocyanates, which stimulate the break down of potential carcinogens.

817 KALE POWER

Curly kale is a neglected superfood full of glucosinolates that help to fight cancer, as well as containing more vitamin C than oranges (vital for skin and hair), along with a healthy dose of fibre.

818 BE A SMOKE-FREE ZONE

Within weeks of stopping smoking, the circulation improves. Your skin will look better, oxygen levels in your blood will return to normal, your lungs will start to get rid of mucus so breathing becomes easier, and you will have a lot more energy.

819 LUTEIN FOR HEALTHY EYES

Many people suffer from long-sightedness, cataracts, glaucoma and other eye problems as they age. To keep your eyes healthy, increase your level of lutein – available in vegetables such as carrots, broccoli, spinach, Brussels sprouts and kale. Lutein can decrease the risk of cataracts and macular degeneration.

820 GUARD AGAINST WINTER FLU

As you get older, you have an increased susceptibility to colds and flu, especially those brought on by a seasonal shift from summer to autumn. Be prepared by taking extra steps to support your immune system with the herbal remedy echinacea, but don't forget to get a winter flu immunization too.

821 EAT WATERCRESS TO FIGHT CANCER

Watercress has just been declared the latest superfood in the battle to protect cells from changes that lead to cancer. It is also a better source of vitamins C, B1, calcium, magnesium and zinc than many other vegetables, all of which are needed for healthy skin and eyes.

822 HELP HOT FLUSHES

Add lots of phyto-oestrogen vegetables to your diet such as kale, fennel, yams, and all types of beans. Try using a red clover supplement that is high in isoflavones, which are thought to reduce menopausal symptoms and improve cholesterol levels.

823 STAY STRONG WITH VITAMIN D

An essential vitamin that requires synthesis from sunlight to turn it into an active form, vitamin D can help with back pain and aching joints, and slow the progression of osteoporosis. It is found in milk and fish such as salmon and sardines, so include plenty of these in your diet.

824 THE GARLIC CURE

For a long time, garlic has been known as one of nature's best remedies. It can lower blood pressure and cholesterol, and help your heart. In addition, it boosts the immune system as well as protect the body from viral and bacterial infections.

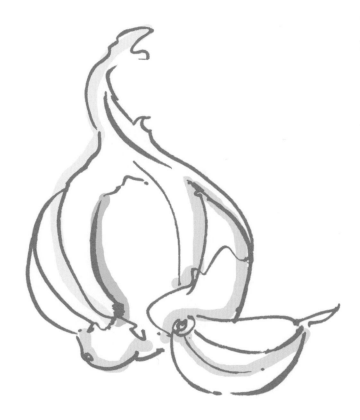

825 NATURAL HRT

Black cohosh and flaxseed are two supplements that can help regulate your hormones during menopause and counter common symptoms, as both are high in phyto-oestrogens. Black cohosh has a long history of being beneficial for PMS/PMT symptoms, arthritis and muscle pain, and night sweats. Many doctors recommend a three-month treatment only. Flaxseed is claimed to lower the risk of certain cancers, cardiovascular disease and hypertension. Cholesterol levels may also decrease and it may help aches and pains.

826 KEEP YOUR BONES HEALTHY

To prevent osteoporosis, which can cause curvature of the spine and back and leg pain, ask your doctor if you should take a daily calcium tablet. Choose juice, water and foods that are specially fortified with calcium, and make sure you get sufficient calcium from your diet in foods such as milk, cheese, yogurt and dark green leafy vegetables. Post-menopausal women need 1200 to 1500 mg of calcium daily.

827 AVOID ALCOHOL AND CAFFEINE

Eliminating alcohol, caffeine and spicy foods from your diet can reduce the hot-flush symptoms of menopause. In addition, caffeine can cause insomnia and lead to the greater loss of calcium from the body.

828 TAKE SOYA TO PREVENT SYMPTOMS

In Japan, where soya-based foods are eaten daily, women are only one-third as likely to report menopausal symptoms as women in the West. The phyto-oestrogens in soya help regulate the hormone system, so to prevent symptoms, start taking soya milk in your coffee or include tofu in your diet.

829 STAND TALL

People of both sexes and all races typically shrink about 1 cm (½ inch) in height every ten years after they reach the age of 40 and even more after the age of 70. Physical activity, a good diet and treating osteoporosis and muscle weakness can help reduce this loss of height.

830 KEEP YOUR BONES HEALTHY

To prevent osteoporosis, which can cause curvature of the spine, back and leg pain, ask your doctor if you should take a daily calcium tablet after the age of 40. Choose juice, water and foods that are specially fortified with calcium, and make sure you get sufficient calcium through your diet – eating such foods as milk, cheese, yogurt and dark green leafy vegetables. Post-menopausal women need 1200 to 1500 mg of calcium daily.

boost your energy

831 GET A NATURAL HIGH

For a burst of natural energy, avoid known stimulants like caffeine and alcohol and opt for the herbal stimulant guarana. Sold in health shops in powder or syrup form, it is thought to increase mental attentiveness, fight fatigue and increase stamina.

832 TIRED OF BEING TIRED

For instant energy, carry a packet of seeds or nuts in your handbag. They contain high levels of the EFAs omega-3 and omega-6, which play a vital role in the maintenance of energy balance and glucose metabolism.

833 BE PREPARED

According to a recent survey, 3.09 pm is the exact time of day when our energy slumps, and people rush to the biscuit tin for a sugar hit. Resist the urge to snack on junk and be ready with fresh fruit, nuts or seeds.

834 FOREGO THE ENERGY SUPPLEMENTS

Guarana, noni juice and yerba tea are all touted as good 'natural' energy boosters, but most of these contain caffeine. Instead, look at your iron and magnesium intake; if these are lower than recommended, increasing them in your diet may aid your flagging energy. Magnesium is found in artichokes, halibut, black beans, almonds and spinach, while good sources for iron are wholegrain cereals, lentils, oatmeal, tofu and dark green leafy vegetables.

835 BE LIKE A MONKEY

Monkeys are known for their high energy, so take a tip from them and eat a banana. They provide potassium, an electrolyte that maintains nerve and muscle function, but levels of it can drop quickly during stress or exercise, as it is lost through sweating.

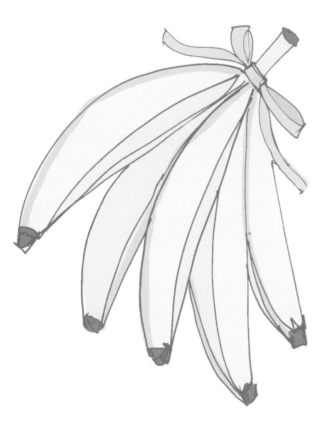

836 OATS FOR ENERGY

Oats are low on the glycaemic index, have lots of fibre and contain the energizing B vitamins, which help transform carbohydrates into usable energy. Choose porridge for an easy supply, but other options are whole grains and brown rice.

837 EAT FOR ENERGY

Fatigue and low energy may be due to a lack of certain nutrients. Look for foods that are strong sources of vitamin B2, magnesium and the antioxidant coenzyme Q10, found in whole grains, legumes, nuts and seafood.

838 ENERGIZE YOUR BODY

A good healthy diet is the single most important way of boosting energy levels. Deficiencies in B vitamins can often be the underlying cause of poor adrenal gland function, which is responsible for energy slumps. Take ginseng and astragalus tea as an afternoon pick-me-up.

weight issues

839 DON'T BLAME YOUR GENES

Genetics account for only 25% of our future body shape. If you need to shift a few pounds, you will have to commit to a lifestyle plan that incorporates a healthy diet, regular exercise and, if you can afford it, some weight-reducing therapies.

840 SPICE IT UP

Hot spicy foods can help the body burn up calories. Using spices like cayenne pepper and chilli elevates the body temperature, which makes the heart beat faster and requires more energy.

841 STOP THE MIDDLE-AGED SPREAD

As we age, increasing amounts of fat tissue can be deposited around the abdominal organs, and the proportion of body fat may increase by as much as 30%. Reducing your consumption of calories, especially those derived from fat, will help.

842 STAY SLIM FOR LONGER LIFE

Carrying excess baggage around may increase the risk of dying young by as much as 50%. Overweight women are more likely to have high blood pressure, high cholesterol and some cancers. Don't rely on unhealthy slimming diets to keep your weight down: go for lots of fresh food and regular exercise instead.

843 EXERCISE YOURSELF SLIM

Our bodies change as we grow older, and an older body is often a fatter body. As well as a nutritionally complete diet that is low in calories and fat, exercise will help shift those pounds by speeding up your metabolism and burning up extra calories – and it will tone up your muscles too.

844 MUNCH ON NEGATIVE CALORIES

If you want to snack on something that won't pile on the weight, try a stick of celery: it takes more energy to digest celery than it contains in calories.

845 MAINTAIN WEIGHT FOR BETTER HEALTH

After the age of 40, it is natural for women to put on weight. They may also discover that it is harder to maintain their weight during the perimenopause, the years leading up to the menopause; on average, women gain about 0.5 kg (1 lb) a year during this time. There is evidence that weight gained at this time also predisposes women to breast cancer, so take preventative action by eating less and burning more calories.

846 FOLLOW THE 80–20 RULE

Drastic food restriction is not the way to a healthier, fitter body. Choose sensible options for 80% of the time, and occasionally relax the rules when you are eating out or have a special celebration. This way you are more likely to stick to good eating principles, and not feel guilty about having the odd treat.

847 A BIGGER BREAKFAST

Nutritionists urge women never to skip breakfast, which ideally should provide about a quarter of your daily calorific needs. People who go without breakfast are more likely to snack on unhealthy food and pile on the calories.

848 EAT YOURSELF THIN

Never be tempted to skip meals in an effort to lose weight. The body depends on eating at regular intervals to keep energy levels and hunger pangs at bay. Starving yourself sends a message to the brain to slow down the metabolism and stop burning calories.

849 KEEP A LOCK ON THE FRIDGE

Late-night snacking on cheese and pasta, which take a long time to digest, will add to your calorie consumption. It will also prevent you drifting into a deep sleep and reduce the amount of time spent in REM, leaving you feeling less rested the following morning.

850 PICK UP A PINEAPPLE

A great fat-busting fruit to eat or juice, fresh pineapple contains the enzyme bromelain, which aids digestion and makes short work of fats and proteins, so it is very good for weight-watchers.

851 SNOOZE DIET

New research has shown that lack of sleep reduces the hormones that regulate the body's muscle-to-fat ratio. So if you want to maximize your metabolism, and keep the pounds off while you are sleeping, aim for a consistent eight hours every night.

852 OLIVES ARE OK

If you need an early evening snack with your glass of wine, choose olives instead of crisps (potato chips), which are calorie-laden. There are loads of different varieties to choose from, and they are all full of great essential fatty acids (EFAs), and contain relatively few calories.

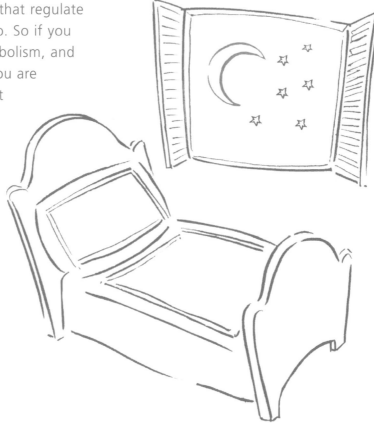

853 INCREASE METABOLIC RATE

Green tea is thought to suppress the ageing process as well as control the ratio of body fat to muscle by promoting thermogenesis – the process whereby heat is created in the body to burn fat, thus increasing the body's metabolic rate.

854 KEEP REGULAR

The longer you leave between meals, the higher your levels of the fat-storing hormone cortisol. Eating regularly every three hours reduces cortisol production, and keeps your metabolism on an even keel.

855 SNACKS ARE GOOD

Small simple meals spaced evenly throughout the day are much better for your metabolism than starving until 6 pm and having one big blow-out meal then. Keep the body sufficiently fuelled by having healthy snacks in-between meals: fruit, rice cakes or a handful of seeds are all good choices.

detoxing

856 DETOX WHILE YOU SLEEP

Release bad toxins through your feet while you do nothing at all but sleep. Sticky patches containing a special mixture of tourmaline, eucalyptus and bamboo vinegar are placed on the soles of the feet to draw out impurities by morning.

857 ONE DAY'S DENIAL

Fasting for 24 hours every now and again is a recognized cleansing process that benefits every part of the body. All organs and the bloodstream get a much-needed rest, during which tissues are purified and given a chance to rejuvenate. Choose a day when you are not busy and can be at home.

858 FLUSH OUT TOXINS

A liver-cleansing detox plan requires you to double the amount of water you drink to flush the toxins out of the system. To help rid the body of detoxicity overload, up your intake of herbal teas and fresh vegetable and fruit juices.

859 GO ORGANIC FOR DETOX DIET

Even if you decide to do only a 24-hour rejuvenating detox, you must always buy organic fruit and vegetables otherwise you will be replacing some of the toxins you are trying to get rid of with dangerous pesticide residues – and thus defeating the purpose of the detox.

860 RAW IS BEST

Food in its natural raw state is full of active vitamins, minerals, proteins and life-enhancing enzymes. Cooking destroys all enzymes and makes up to 85% of nutrients unavailable. The healthiest option is raw food, which will cleanse and rejuvenate the body, making the hair more lustrous, the eyes clearer and the body systems more efficient.

861 SIP ON A LEMON

Lemon is a very good oil for detoxifying and stimulating a sluggish system, which can help with weight loss. Rosemary is also recommended, as it can help promote clarity of thought and improve concentration.

862 DETOXIFY THE BODY

Cutting down on processed foods that contain large amounts of sugar, salt and additives, as well as other toxins like alcohol, caffeine and nicotine, will allow your body to cleanse itself, leaving you feeling more energized and youthful. It enlivens your digestive body system and cleanses your liver and kidneys.

863 NATUROPATHY

This is a detoxing therapy based on the idea that stress, pollution, lack of sleep and exercise and a poor diet all result in a build-up of toxins. Non-invasive treatments such as massage, hydrotherapy, herbal remedies and diet overhaul are used to return the body to a state of balance. See www.naturopaths.org.uk.

864 DOCTOR'S ORDERS

Anyone considering a detox should consult their doctor first. Detoxing is not recommended for anyone with diabetes, liver problems, gut ulcers or who is on warfarin therapy.

865 JUICY FRUITS

Juicing is one of the easiest ways to consume fresh fruit and vegetables on a daily basis. Choose food that is as fresh as possible, and always drink the juice straight away, as oxidization starts within minutes, and the benefits of vitamins, minerals and antioxidants will be lost. Carrots and apples are among the best ingredients to choose.

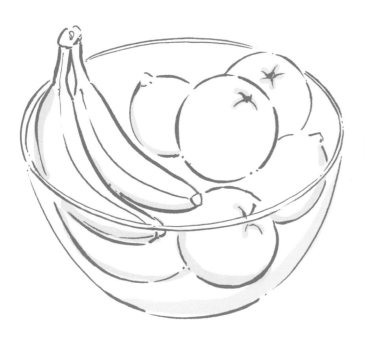

866 GET A LOAD OF NUTRIENTS

To obtain the most from fresh fruit and vegetables when you are juicing, use virtually the whole item of food. Use organic products and throw in the leaves, the tops and outer skins, as well as the skins and stems for maximum nutrients.

867 THE POWER OF ENZYMES

Enzymes are special proteins that act as catalysts to jump-start almost every aspect of a healthy body. They assist in fighting ageing, weight loss, lowering cholesterol and detoxifying the body. Cooking destroys some of their power.

good habits

868 BALANCE BLOOD SUGAR LEVELS

Glowing skin, boundless energy and a steady body weight can all be achieved by keeping blood sugar levels stabilized. Eat five small meals throughout the day, to benefit from balanced glucose levels.

869 EAT UP TO LOOK YOUNGER

Studies at London's Institute of Optimum
Nutrition have shown that women who are
consistently underweight and follow highly
restrictive diets are always deficient in a
wide range of vitamins and minerals and
age far more quickly. Stick to three meals
a day for optimum health.

870 A MINIMUM OF FIVE

In Britain, the government recommends
five portions of fruit and vegetables a day
to provide the right amount of nutrients
and antioxidants to keep you fit and
healthy. Australia recommends seven
portions a day, and France ten! So eat
more if you can.

871 DISCOVER THE GI INDEX

The rate at which different
carbohydrate foods release glucose
into the bloodstream affects energy levels.
The glycaemic index is a ranking system
that measures food values from 0–100.
It does not relate to calories, but to how
quickly sugar affects blood glucose levels.

872 STOP AT 7 PM

Do your body a favour and breakfast like
a king, lunch like a prince and dine like
a pauper. If you make the last meal of
the day the smallest, and eat it early in
the evening, food is not left sitting in the
stomach overnight when your metabolism
has slowed right down.

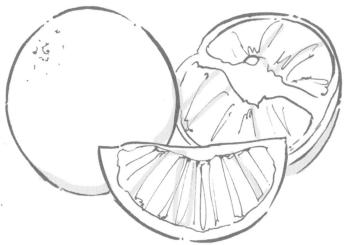

873 BROWN IS BEST

As a general food-shopping rule, stick to brown foods if you have the choice. Nearly all white foods have been highly processed (to make them white) and provide fewer nutrients and more sugar. Brown bread, pasta, flour and pitta bread are better for you than their white equivalents.

874 CHOOSE ORGANIC

Wherever possible, choose organic food. Always wash all fruit and vegetables under the tap before you eat them to remove pesticides that can submit your skin to excess levels of free radicals, leading to wrinkles, saggy skin and loss of elasticity.

875 GOOD FATS MEAN GOOD SKIN

Choosing to eat a diet that is high in essential fats, found in oily fish, avocados, nuts and seeds, will help the appearance and texture of your skin. Include unsaturated fats in your diet to help promote plump, dewy skin.

876 SPLASH OUT ON ORGANIC MILK

Recent studies have shown that organic milk is 50% richer in vitamin E and 75% higher in betacarotene than standard milk – so it will help you fight wrinkle-forming free radicals as well as boost the immune system.

877 FIRM UP WITH FISH

All types of seafood and shellfish contain small amounts of copper, which is used within the body to make collagen fibres and elastin, vital ingredients that mesh together with other proteins to give skin strength and elasticity.

878 EAT UP OR LOSE THE PLOT

If you exist on a highly restricted calorie diet, you run the risk of losing competent brain function. Low levels of magnesium, B vitamins and fatty acids are essential for hormone production and brain function. Without them you can lose the ability to think rationally.

879 LEMON ZESTER

A morning cup of hot water and lemon juice is a great way to start the day. It kickstarts the metabolism after a night's sleep, aids digestion and provides a natural way to cleanse the liver and stomach, as well as providing an excellent source of vitamin C.

880 EAT MEAT FOR ELASTIN

You need to have a regular source of protein in your diet if you want stop wrinkles appearing. Elastin, which keeps skin supple, is a protein, and without a daily supply of protein (the body can't store it) the skin loses some elasticity and wrinkles develop.

881 SNACK ON SEEDS

When an attack of the munchies hits you, a small handful of sunflower seeds is much better for you than a bar of chocolate. Rich in natural compounds that lower cholesterol, seeds are also full of vitamins and minerals that are good for healthy hair and skin.

882 ENERGIZE YOUR METABOLISM

The body needs fuel every few hours to keep blood sugar levels stable, stimulate the metabolism and keep mood swings steady. Avoid eating large rich meals for extra energy because the body has to work hard to digest it, and you will feel tired.

883 GO BANANAS

For a handy and tasty snack, why not try dried banana chips? They are rich in carbohydrates, iron and magnesium and, in addition, contain natural sugars to give your body an energy boost when you're busy. For a more substantial snack, combine with natural yogurt.

884 GOOD FATS MEAN GOOD SKIN

Choosing to eat a diet that is high in unsaturated essential fats, found in oily fish, avocados, nuts and seeds, will help the appearance and texture of your skin. This is because skin cells convert the fats to prostaglandin hormones, which are responsible for making skin soft, smooth and moist.

885 EATING OUT WISELY

Eating out is often associated with the consumption of high-caloric, high-fat and salty foods, but it can be healthy if you are careful about portion control and ask how the food is being prepared and cooked. Choose a starter as your main course if you think the portions will be too large.

886 DRINK WATER FREELY

Keep drinking water, as many people misread thirst signals for hunger signs. The body is made up of nearly 80% water, and a glass of ordinary tap water will benefit nearly every organ in the body, including the skin.

887 NAILS NEED PROTEIN

If your nails are constantly splitting and breaking, it could be a sign that there is a lack of protein in your diet. Rich sources are meat, poultry, fish and soy. A protein formula varnish, specifically designed to strengthen nails, will also help.

nutritional no-nos

888 FLUSHED WITH BOOZE

Drinking alcohol excessively will dehydrate your system, and leave skin prematurely aged. Too much alcohol in the system dilates small blood vessels in the skin, which causes increased blood flow near the skin's surface. Over time, these blood vessels can become permanently damaged, causing a flushed appearance.

889 BAD SUGAR BLUES

We all know it's bad for us, but new research has conclusively proved that too much white sugar will cause premature ageing, particularly around the eye area where skin is fragile and prone to wrinkles.

890 BOOZE IS BAD FOR YOU

Limit alcohol consumption to government guidelines (two to three units a day for women) and try to drink a large glass of water before bed. Alcohol acts as a diuretic and leaves the body dehydrated and skin prematurely old and wrinkled.

891 DUMP BAD FOODS

Refined carbohydrates like cakes, biscuits and sweets, as well as processed ready-made meals, all cause havoc with the healthy working of the mind and body. Our bodies become lethargic and sluggish when processing foods filled with additives and chemical preservatives.

892 AVOID ADDITIVES

Pay attention to labels and look for hidden ingredients with a number like tartrazine E102, and avoid where possible. Colourings and preservatives may interact with the immune system, speeding up the ageing process and possibly promoting carcinogenic changes in cells.

893 CUT OUT CAFFEINE

Never use a cup of tea or coffee as an instant pick-me-up. Caffeine will only provide the body with a short-term boost of energy and the damage it does by dehydrating the system and interfering with its ability to absorb vitamins is much greater.

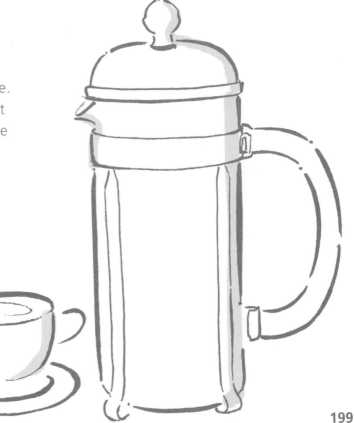

rejuvenate with sleep

894 AVOID STIMULANTS

Lack of sleep can have a negative impact on your body, mind and looks, leading to puffy, tired eyes and dull-looking skin. Avoid stimulants like alcohol, nicotine and caffeine late at night, as these all affect the nervous system and disrupt sleep patterns.

895 GET INTO A ROUTINE

A regular bedtime schedule will help your body to expect sleep at the same time each day. Spend quiet time relaxing in a warm bath infused with a few drops of essential lavender oil to soothe the mind and body and encourage regenerative sleep.

896 SLEEP LIKE AN ITALIAN

Starchy carbohydrates are vital for a healthy body, and an evening meal that has some carbohydrate content can help raise levels of seratonin – a brain chemical that helps control sleep patterns.

897 REGENERATION FUNDS

Scientists know that relaxation is a restorative time for the body, when the body repairs and regenerates itself. It is during its relaxed state that the brain produces 'feel-good molecules', immunity is boosted and the body repairs and forms new tissue.

898 THE HOURS

Sleep between the hours of 10 pm and 6 am if you can. The first four hours are when physical regeneration takes place. The second four bring mental and emotional recharging, so you wake up looking and feeling better.

899 DOWNLOAD FIRST

If you have difficulty nodding off because the worries of the day are still rushing around in your head, get out of bed and write a list of everything that's bothering you, and a to-do list if necessary. Once you have unloaded your brain, you should be able to sink into a regenerative sleep.

900 DRINK UP AT BEDTIME

A hot milky drink at bedtime is good because it contains the amino acid L-tryptophan, a precursor of the sleep-inducing hormones melatonin and serotonin.

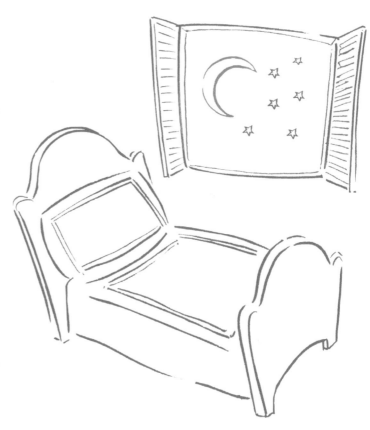

901 NOISE POLLUTION

One of the biggest distractions to getting a good night's sleep is noise. Try to cut out night-time noise when you go to bed, even if it means wearing ear plugs. Sleep is a regenerative time, but you need some uninterrupted hours for your body to restore itself.

902 SIMULATE MELATONIN

Ageing can blur your waking and sleeping patterns, but numerous researchers have found that the hormone melatonin can enhance longevity, promote deep and restful sleep, slow cell damage and ageing, as well as support the immune system and improve energy levels. Enhance your natural levels of melatonin by always going to sleep in the dark.

903 NOD OFF NATURALLY

The herb valerian has been used in traditional sleep remedies for hundreds of years. It is thought to relieve anxiety and to aid the induction of sleep in a natural and non-addictive way.

904 FIND THE RIGHT POSITION

Learn to sleep on your back – it's the best position for relaxing and it allows all your internal organs to rest properly.

905 REPAIR THE BRAIN

According to research by Princeton University for the World Health Organization, missing out on sleep may cause the brain to stop producing new cells and can negatively affect the part of the brain called the hippocampus, which is responsible for forming memories. Middle-aged people should get seven hours a night – you know you are getting enough when you wake spontaneously without an alarm clock.

906 SWEET FRESH SLEEP

Good sleep comes in a room that has a window ajar. Unexpected odours disrupt sleep patterns, increasing the heart rate and quickening brain waves. Sprinkle some heliotropine, a vanilla-almond fragrance on your pillow, to help promote a good night's sleep.

907 PILLOW PRESSURE

Reduce stress and tension by resting on a thermal neck pillow that can be heated up in the microwave. The heat generated by the pillow penetrates the tense neck muscles, soothing away aches and pains and relieving headaches and those oh-so ageing frowns.

908 COPY THE CONTINENTALS

The Mediterranean habit of a siesta has enormous health benefits as we get older. A 'disco nap' between the hours of 3 pm and 5 pm, where you take off your clothes and get properly into bed, will leave you with more energy, alertness and enthusiasm for the evening ahead.

909 LULL WITH LAVENDER

Place a small lavender-filled pillow in your bed to promote a restful night's sleep. The herb is thought to reduce levels of anxiety and promote general feelings of wellbeing.

wellbeing therapies

910 SCULPT A FLAT TUMMY

Regular massage of your own tummy with essential oils will kick start the lymphatic drainage system, and physically break up fatty deposits stored there. Use the palm of your hand in flat circular motions, and rub gently to avoid damage to essential organs.

911 CALMING FRAZZLED NERVES

If jittery nerves get the better of you in a social situation, and you find yourself blushing easily, try stimulating the acupoint at the top of the crown of your head to restore emotional balance and relieve anxiety.

912 THE IMPORTANCE OF BREATHING

Good rhythmic breathing is something that needs to be practised. Regular controlled breathing will strengthen the respiratory system, reduce the chaos in your head and soothe the nervous system, allowing you to feel inner calm and in control of your life.

913 BE ALTERNATIVE

If you're interested in complementary medicine as an alternative to rushing off to the GP, you may want to search out a good naturopath. Their skills combine homeopathy, herbalism and nutrition. A good practitioner will investigate the underlying problems of your symptoms, not just provide a quick-fix prescription.

914 SCENT TO HELP

The right essential oils can help to relieve tension and de-stress. Try lavender, chamomile, geranium, spearmint and peppermint, either added to your bath water for a relaxing soak, or inhaled by placing a few drops on a cotton wool pad.

915 EXTREMELY CHILLING

Hydrotherapy treatments can be carried out successfully at home rather than in a salon. Extremes of water temperature are used to jump-start the system, stimulate the lymph and blood circulation, and strengthen the immune system, so you are less susceptible to passing infections.

916 GOOD VIBRATIONS

The simple action of stimulating nerve endings in your head with an electric or a manual head-tingling massager will ease away head and neck pain, and help relax stiff shoulders and tension headaches – all of which cause faces to tighten (leading to wrinkles) and frown lines to form.

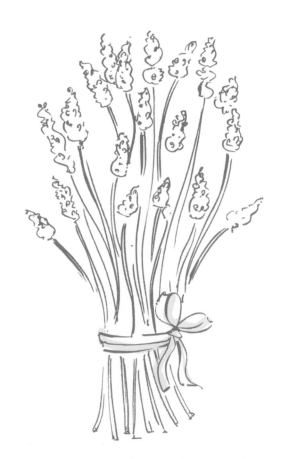

917 OIL THERAPY

Aromatherapy is a system of caring for the body with essential plant oils that are sourced from around the world and used for their therapeutic and healing properties. The essential oils can be added to a bath, massaged through the skin, inhaled directly or used as a compress. The therapy can relieve pain, care for the skin and alleviate tension.

918 RUB AWAY HEADACHES

When massaging in hand cream, pay particular attention to the skin between your thumb and index finger. This is a pressure point used in traditional Chinese medicine to stimulate the lymphatic system and ease headaches.

919 SOAK IN THE DEAD SEA

Plan a trip to the Dead Sea in Israel to soak up the healing powers of the salt and minerals, or purchase Dead Sea salts. Skin will benefit from the medicinal properties of the salt and mud, leaving it looking better outwardly and with a greater elasticity.

920 TRY HOMEOPATHY FOR OSTEOARTHRITIS

There is promising evidence that homeopathy is an effective treatment for the degenerative joint condition osteoarthritis. See a practitioner for the correct remedy and dosage, which will stimulate the body's curative powers to overcome symptoms during illness.

921 COMPLEMENTARY TREATMENTS

There are many alternative treatments and therapies on offer, with practitioners providing a host of remedies for all sorts of problems. Despite a lack of scientific proof, more and more people are convinced that an integrated approach to health and beauty will provide the best results.

922 CELEBRITY DETOX

Many Hollywood celebs favour the Chinese treatment known as 'cupping', which uses heated cups to draw out toxins. It relieves muscle and joint pain and treats digestive problems. Go to www.acupuncture.org.uk for more details.

923 THE WHOLE PICTURE

Holistic therapists take the whole person into account when diagnosing, so you have to be prepared to look honestly at your daily routines of food, exercise, supplements, drugs, sleeping patterns and day-to-day relationships if you want to get the best from the treatment.

924 EARLY-MORNING SHOWER

Alternate the temperature of your shower water between warm for 2 minutes and freezing cold for 30 seconds, and repeat several times. Try not to hold your breath during the cold part, as it will interfere with your body's adaptation to the cold, and finish by splashing cold water onto your face. Your complexion will tingle, and energy levels will be increased throughout the day.

925 SOAK IN SEAWEED

Look out for seaweed-infused bath products. A warm soak in therapeutic marine algae can reduce tension, boost circulation and help to expel toxins from the body.

926 HEAD FOR INDIA

Back and shoulder pain caused by hours slumped over a computer will manifest itself as tense expressions and a face full of frown lines. A traditional Indian head massage (*champissage*) uses deep thumb and finger pressure, to improve blood flow, release tension and create an enhanced state of relaxation.

927 ASK FOR ACUPUNCTURE

Used to rebalance the vital life force 'chi' of the body, acupuncture involves the insertion of tiny needles into specific pulse points to stimulate a blockage of energy. It is used to treat headaches, back pain, osteoarthritis, IBS, skin complaints, depression and addiction.

928 HOMEOPATHY HELPS

Scientific tests about this form of treatment have proved inconclusive, but there is much anecdotal evidence testifying to its success. Treatment is tailored to the individual, and a practitioner prescribes tiny does of highly diluted plant or mineral extracts in the form of tinctures taken on the tongue.

929 AYURVEDIC AS AN AID

Ayurveda is an ancient Indian folk medicine that incorporates a large variety of treatments including massage, nutrition and exercise to restore and revitalize the body. It utilizes the curative properties of plants, herbs and essential oils to improve the skin's health and relieve the stress, tension and emotion of daily life.

930 BETTER WITH BIO

Useful for relaxation and to relieve stress, bio-healing is a complementary medicine that requires the patient to have faith in the process. Without touching, a bio-energy healer can draw negative energy out of the body and channel positive energy in, while their hands hover just above the body.

931 DETOX WITH PRESSURE

The Chinese method of acupressure combines massage and acupuncture, and works by releasing blocked energy located in the meridian lines that run through the body. Using only the thumbs, energy paths are unblocked and toxins are eliminated.

932 HOT STONE HEALING

The Chinese have been using hot stones to relieve muscular pain for thousands of years. In hot stone therapy (known as geothermotherapy), water-heated basalt stones are placed at key points along the spine. The direct heat and deep massage increase blood flow, relax muscles and support detoxification from the liver and kidneys – and it's very, very relaxing.

933 CRYSTAL HEALING

Healers claim that every living organism has a 'vibrational energy system', which includes chakras, subtle bodies and meridians. By using the appropriate crystals, the healer can fine-tune an energy system, rebalance energies and improve wellbeing.

934 CONSIDER COLOUR THERAPY

Chromotherapy is an alternative medicine method where a trained therapist uses colour and light to balance emotional, spiritual or physical energies. It is often combined with hydrotherapy and aromatherapy to bring about an emotional reaction.

935 DEEP-SEA TREATMENT

Thalassotherapy refers to a variety of treatments that involve ocean-derived ingredients like seaweed, mud and sea minerals, all of which are saturated in mineral salts, trace elements and amino acids. Each type of treatment is designed to tone, moisturize and revitalize the body and skin. Nutrients from the sea transfer to the body when placed on the skin, and circulation is improved.

936 REFLEXOLOGY

In this holistic practice, which deals with all aspects of the mind and body, the practitioner uses the thumb and fingers of the hand on certain parts of the hands or feet that correspond to our internal organs. Reflexology stimulates blocked meridians to promote general wellbeing and ease specific complaints.

relaxing & de-stressing

937 CD MEANS CALM DOWN

To reduce stress or that panicky feeling of having far too much to do, buy a hypnotherapy CD. Lie down and listen to a calming voice, letting all your worries drift away and reducing the chaos in your mind – your face will relax too!

938 GET HELP

Seek professional help if you feel consumed by anger, jealousy or guilt. These emotions are 'poisonous' to a healthy mind and body, and could eventually lead to stress-related illnesses.

939 GOAL-ORIENTATED VISUALIZATION

Sit quietly for 5 minutes a day in a calm meditative state where you visualize yourself in any situation of warmth and happiness to get rid of stress, tension and anxiety – all of which cause headaches and frown lines.

940 ACCENTUATE THE POSITIVE

Cognitive behavioural therapy (CBT) believes that negative attitudes and beliefs are unhealthy modes of thinking that have been learned over a long time. It challenges this way of thinking and encourages you to take a more positive and assertive view.

941 BAN NEGATIVE WORDS

Words like 'can't', 'won't' and 'shouldn't' all have negative connotations that make you think in a pessimistic way. Take a more positve approach. Studies have shown that optimists are healthier people who have higher levels of antibodies and greater energy.

942 GO DEEPER WITHIN

Shut off from the material world and practise meditation. Sitting cross-legged for just 10 minutes a day, listening to your own breath, each inhale and exhale, and letting go of your emotional baggage will calm a stressed mind and body and give you better perspective.

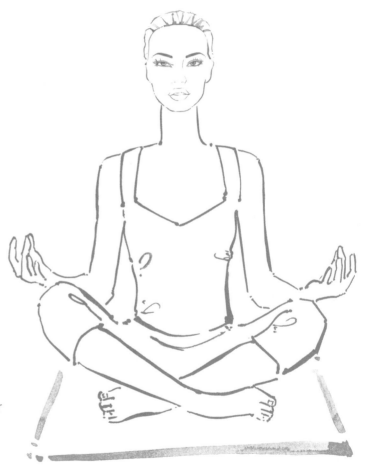

943 AN END TO CONFLICT

Arguments and hostility lead to an endless release of the stress hormone cortisol. The hormone raises blood sugar, and high levels of excess cortisol lead to excess fat being deposited on the body, particularly around the tummy area. No one can avoid conflict completely, but investigate some cognitive behavioural techniques to reduce the negative feelings that conflict brings.

944 MAKE TIME FOR YOU

Spending time quietly alone, where you can empty your mind of all your thoughts, learn to focus and begin to feel a calm awareness of the world around you, will provide physical and mental health benefits, as long as you do it regularly.

945 CHANTING FOR THE INNER YOU

Meditative chanting can diminish all negative feelings such as anger, envy, boredom and greed. The process encourages a kind of inner happiness brought about by the transcendental sound vibrations of chanting.

946 GET A FURRY FRIEND

As stress-busters go, this is one of the nicest ways to lift your mood and relieve stress, as long as you're not allergic to dogs! Bad moods disappear with a furry puppy on your lap – they provide companionship and unconditional love, and they encourage you to get outdoors.

947 TAKE SOME TIME OUT

Book a week away from it all at a country retreat, spa or religious centre, where you can take advantage of complementary therapies and treatments. You will experience the benefits of relaxation, develop inner strength and refresh your mind and body away from daily stresses.

948 GET IN TOUCH WITH YOURSELF

Become more self-aware and get in touch with your inner feelings so that you can identify different emotions. An easy visualization technique is to blank the mind and think only of blue sky and a white sandy beach. Imagine you are in that sunny situation and how it feels.

949 ISOLATE YOUR MUSCLES

Get into the habit of using relaxation techniques such as progressive muscle relaxation, where you tense, hold for 10 seconds then release each muscle group one by one. Used regularly, it can improve your immune system and coping skills, as well as significantly reducing the likelihood of a heart attack.

950 STRENGTHEN YOUR CORE

Pilates is a slow and controlled set of movements that helps to improve coordination and provide greater awareness of each part of the body as you focus on breathing techniques and postural alignment. By learning to relax more deeply, you can reduce stress in all areas of your life.

951 TOO MUCH INFORMATION

Most of us are overstimulated. Resolve to not watch TV or buy any newspapers for a week. Turn off your mobile for at least a few hours every day and limit home time on email to the weekends.

952 RESOLVE TO RELAX

Clean your body and your mind, and let yourself have a few minutes of uninterrupted time in a relaxing bath. Add skin-softening milk, and let yourself drift off, letting the problems of the day float away with the bubbles.

think yourself younger

953 PRACTISE MEMORY GAMES

Keep the brain healthy by exercising your failing memory. Directly after a social occasion, re-live the event in your head – the plot of the movie or play, the costumes or set. Or if you were at a party, try to recall individual details about the people you met. Use visual clues to help you remember – the stranger and more unusual, the more likely it is you will be able to recall the associated information later on.

954 BE A MULTITASKER

According to a study at Trinity College, Dublin, juggling many tasks at once helps to keep your mind young and active. As we age, we challenge ourselves mentally less and less, and the effort involved in keeping several things to the forefront of your mind at once exercises the brain.

955 USE IT OR LOSE IT

Keep challenging yourself mentally to learn a new skill, take up a new hobby or read more books. Research has shown that brain cells need to be exercised in the same way that the physical body does to keep fit and healthy.

956 BINGO BOOSTS BRAIN CELLS

Keeping the brain mentally active is thought to help maintain mental alertness. Bingo players have been found to be faster and more accurate in tests than non-bingo players, and mental agility is believed to stave off depression and degenerative brain disease.

957 KEEP NOTE OF YOUR FIVE SENSES

Practise a daily mental workout to avoid sluggish thinking and memory loss; mental decline with old age is not inevitable if the brain remains busy. Make up your own exercises to strengthen all five senses – sight, sound, smell, taste and touch – and keep a record to note down week-by-week enhancements of each.

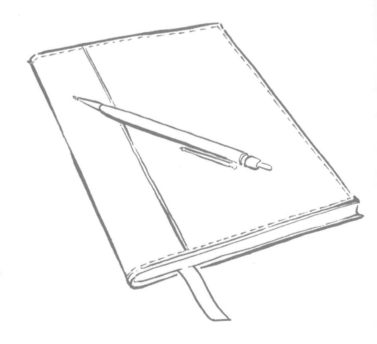

958 FOCUS YOUR MIND ON A HOBBY

Our brains naturally start slowing down at the age of 30. However, new studies show that people of any age can train their brains to be faster and, in effect, younger. Experts say that any hobby that closely engages your focus and is strongly rewarding will kick your brain into learning mode and notch it up.

959 CHEW GUM FOR MEMORY

Studies show that chewing gum can improve long-term and working memory. The chewing action increases the heart rate, improving the delivery of oxygen and nutrients to the brain, and triggers the release of insulin, which may stimulate memory.

960 STAY CONNECTED

Make a concerted effort to keep up-to-date with technological advances. Get an iPod and download some current music tracks or podcasts, or log onto YouTube or MySpace. Don't try to compete with younger people – just keep abreast of trends and make sure you know what they're talking about.

961 CROSS WORDS

Research has shown that keeping the mind agile is just as important as keeping fit in the battle to stay young. A lazy brain needs exercising in the same way that the body does. Try to do a crossword puzzle or play a game of Sudoku every day to stimulate brain cells and keep them active and healthy. Other claimed benefits include the delay or prevention of Alzheimer's disease.

962 STOP BRAIN-CELL DECLINE

After the age of 35, brain cells die off at a rate of 100,000 per day and are not replaced. Meditation can reduce this decaying process as it changes the vibratory make-up of the mind.

963 SET GOALS

If you want to make changes in your life, it helps to set achievable goals. There are no quick fixes to roll back the ravages of time, but changing bad habits and looking at lifestyle changes will give you a positive outlook for the future.

964 HAVE AN ADVENTURE

Remember when the world seemed like such an exciting place and you couldn't wait to explore it? There's no need to lose that feeling just because you're a little bit older. Book an adventure holiday, such as a trek in another country, or go somewhere you've never been before. Eat the local food and immerse yourself in the culture – you will go a long way towards stimulating your mind and helping yourself to feel active and youthful.

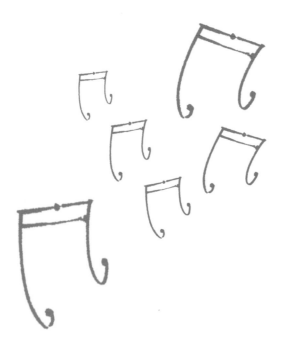

965 A DIFFERENT PATH

Changing your daily habits slightly will help you keep a fresh perspective. For example, vary the route you take to walk to work, and take some time to notice the different surroundings. If you drive a car, take a longer route occasionally, or if you always have lunch at a specific time, take it an hour later.

966 SPEAK IN TONGUES

Learning a second language forces your brain to switch tracks continuously, which is one of the most mentally demanding things you can do. It's particularly effective for honing the frontal lobes – the brain's mind manager – which generally shrink with age.

967 GET EDUCATED

Many of us who would like to learn a new language or master a musical instrument are put off by the fact that we will not be as 'quick' as we were when we were kids. But research has proved that the greater our education – no matter when we achieved it – the more likely we are to live long and fulfilled lives.

968 LEARN TO LOVE WHAT YOU HATE

Taking up a task or skill you've never particularly enjoyed is a good way to address lazy thought patterns. For example, if you've never enjoyed history, try memorizing some facts, or if you have a block about maths, exercise accounting skills. Going against type will invigorate the mind and prevent predictable ways of thinking.

969 SCARE YOURSELF SILLY

Everyone slips into safe routines and situations. To keep young, you need to be aware that this may not help you grow and develop – which is important at any age. Try doing something that frightens you a little – it could be as challenging as parachuting or bungee-jumping, or simply having a weekend away on your own.

970 COGNITIVE POWERS OF THE FUTURE

Ampakines, a class of drugs that enhances learning, memory and concentration, are being developed and also aid sufferers of Alzheimer's, Parkinson's and other age-related mental disabilities.

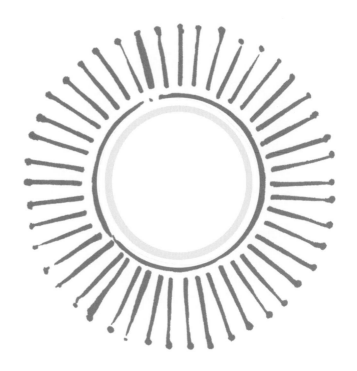

mood boosters

971 KEEP A SUNNY OUTLOOK

Don't let yourself become overanxious to the point that fears and worries dominate your whole life. A worried mind is not at peace and it will deplete energy levels, which you need to maintain youthfulness.

972 PUT ON A HAPPY FACE

Nothing is more attractive than someone with a happy smile – it makes you look young, fun and carefree. Research has shown that people who practise fake smiling actually end up feeling happier as a result – just as those who practise frowning feel more depressed.

973 THINK HAPPY

Learn to be happy within yourself, and not to compare your life, looks or financial situation with others. No amount of surgery, needles or scalpels will change the way you feel inside. An optimistic nature, a network of supportive friends and some feeling of control over your life are some of the most important things for graceful, stress-free ageing.

974 IMPROVE MOOD WITH SELENIUM

When US Department of Agriculture (USDA) researchers fed young men a diet that contained 220 mcg of the mineral selenium per day (the average American diet has 40 to 60 mcg), the men reported feeling elated, clearheaded, confident and energetic.

975 GIVE BLOOD

Rolling up your sleeve and donating blood to help save someone else's life will remind you that there are others more needy than you. You will also benefit from having your blood pressure, pulse and haemoglobin levels checked.

976 BRAIN FOOD

People who eat breakfast are happier, and studies have proved that early morning food has beneficial effects on mental and physical functions. The body needs to refuel after sleep, and breakfast eaters have higher concentration levels in the morning.

977 BEAUTY FROM WITHIN

Comparing yourself to supermodels, movie stars or even the yummy mummy on the school run is not a good idea. Stop worrying what other people think of you. Real beauty is about confidence and not about achieving a certain size of figure or attaining wealth. Start feeling good about yourself and you will begin to radiate an inner beauty.

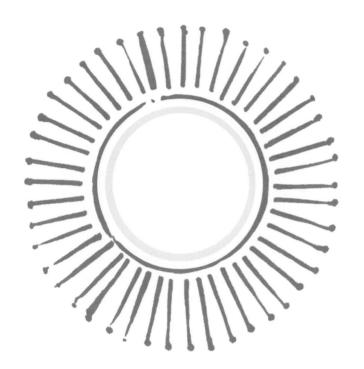

979 GRUMPY OLD GALS

We all make excuses about why we eat the wrong foods, don't have enough time to exercise and drink too much alcohol. The truth is we do have the power to change the things we dislike about our lives. A commitment to making small changes can lead to a healthier and more fulfilling life.

980 FOCUS ON THE POSITIVE

Emotion researchers have discovered that as people get older, they experience fewer negative emotions and report better control over their emotions – they also tend to enhance positive memories and diminish negative ones. Mirror this 'positivity effect' by dismissing every negative thought that comes your way.

978 GOOD MORNING

Be happier by getting up earlier in the morning. Researchers from the University of California have found that early-morning light raised levels of luteinizing hormone (LH) by up to 70%. This hormone can help to build muscle, cut fat and elevate mood.

981 THE KARMA OF KINDNESS

Being kind to others has positive health benefits both physically and mentally. A rush of euphoria, followed by a longer period of calm, is known as the 'helper's high', which can trigger feel-good endorphins into the body and help ease depression.

982 BE HAPPY-GO-LUCKY

People who maximize opportunities, are open to new experiences and act instinctively are more likely to create their own luck, increase their self-esteem and generate a positive energy.

983 YOUNG AT HEART

Make sure your social group of friends includes some who are much younger. Having young friends who have a less cynical and more optimistic approach to life will keep energy levels high, and make you feel and look younger.

984 GRAB A LITTLE LOVING

Feelings of love and trust between a couple and a healthy sex life have been scientifically proved to make you feel good all over. Good sex releases endorphins in the brain that create an overall level of contentment. It can also act as a natural tranquillizer that calms you down and promotes good sleep, as well as making you feel fit, healthy and younger. So what's stopping you?

985 WATCH A WEEPY

Research has shown that it's good to have a good cry now and again. Tears appear to reduce tension, remove toxins and increase the body's ability to heal itself. After an outburst of tears, the body is flooded with oxygen, which triggers the release of feel-good hormones in the brain.

986 FIND SOMEONE TO CUDDLE

Research shows that cuddling decreases levels of stress hormones and boosts levels of serotonin in the brain. Regular cuddles can stimulate the production of feel-good endorphins and oxytocin, making you feel and look happier and younger.

987 BEAT THE BLUES

If you're prone to depression take preventative action with a course of the herbal remedy St John's Wort (hypericum). In clinical trials it has proved successful in helping to lift mild depression and calm anxiety. It's a good idea to consult a health professional first though.

988 HAVE A GOOD CHAT

Interacting with others can bring about a deep sense of relaxation and happiness for women. Recent studies have proven that the act of talking triggers a flood of chemicals, which (scientists say) give women a rush similar to that felt by heroin addicts on a high!

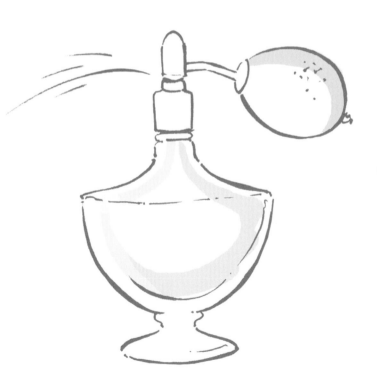

989 FALL IN LOVE

Maybe easier to say than to do, but falling in love produces a surge of feel-good endorphins in the brain (dopamine, norepinephrine and phenylethylamine), which are responsible for uncontrollable feelings of euphoria. This huge chemical hit inside the brain gives you flushed cheeks and a racing heart, and will make you look and feel five years younger. If the real deal proves elusive, cultivate crushes and flirt – it will still trigger that rush of endorphins and you'll have lots of fun in the process!

990 SMELLS TO LIVE FOR

Make yourself feel extra special by spritzing on a new scent or using a room spray or scented candles in the home. Fragrances can be very powerful memory triggers, taking you back to a special time and place where you can relive happy memories. They are also relaxants.

981 NURTURE YOUR RELATIONSHIP

Studies have shown that people who are married or in a loving relationship reduce their risk of illness by 50%. Married couples live longer, are less stressed and are said to have fewer heart attacks than single people.

982 THE SOUND OF MUSIC

If you're feeling blue, turn on your favourite CD, and have your own private karaoke session! The physical act of loud singing, combined with the rhythmic breathing it entails, will make you feel much better about yourself.

983 HAVE A GIGGLE

Laughter may be the best medicine after all, as it has been shown to increase blood flow by more than 20% – similar to that of aerobic activity. So a good laugh at a funny movie may help fight infections, ease pain and control diabetes. It has also been shown that people who laugh daily have stronger immune systems and live longer.

984 DOWN AND DIRTY

Spend an afternoon potting and pruning to put yourself into a good mood and relieve tension. Reconnecting with the earth and nature has a calming effect on stress levels, and strenuous digging will give you a fabulous rosy glow.

985 BECAUSE YOU'RE WORTH IT

In being great providers, women often lose sight of their own needs. It's important to make time in the week to do something for yourself – stay in contact with friends, go and watch a movie or take up a new hobby. Finding something that makes you happy will increase your confidence and general feelings of wellbeing.

986 EAT A HAPPY MEAL

Food can directly affect the neurotransmitter chemicals in your brain responsible for maintaining an elevated mood. For the best mood boost, combine lean proteins with complex carbohydrates. Ease up on saturated fats and convenience foods.

987 SEIZE THE DAY

Make every day count, and at the end of it you will feel more content and peaceful within yourself. Wear new clothes, drink that bottle of champagne and don't save your special perfume for best.

988 SLOW DOWN

Living at breakneck speed and using stimulants like caffeine and alcohol to boost levels of adrenaline is very damaging to the body. It lowers immunity and weakens the digestive system, as well as triggering mood swings. Make time for yourself each day to contemplate life.

999 DON'T WORRY, BE HAPPY

Stress and worry cause frowning, and over time the muscles in the face actually conform to that movement and stress wrinkles are formed. Be aware of your stress levels and try to vary your facial expressions during the day – laughter is both a good stress buster and a great facial exercise.

1000 GET CREATIVE WITH SCENT

Sweet-smelling perfume is thought to help boost creativity and encourage problem solving. Dab your favourite scent on your wrists and collarbones, but not behind your ears as the oily skin there interferes with the fragrance.

1001 SAY IT WITH FLOWERS

Research from Texas A&M University found that flowers and plants could help to raise spirits and improve levels of creativity and feelings of happiness. A few bunches of fragrant flowers can be enough to scent your home and lift your mood for days.

INDEX